The Aromatherapy Kitchen

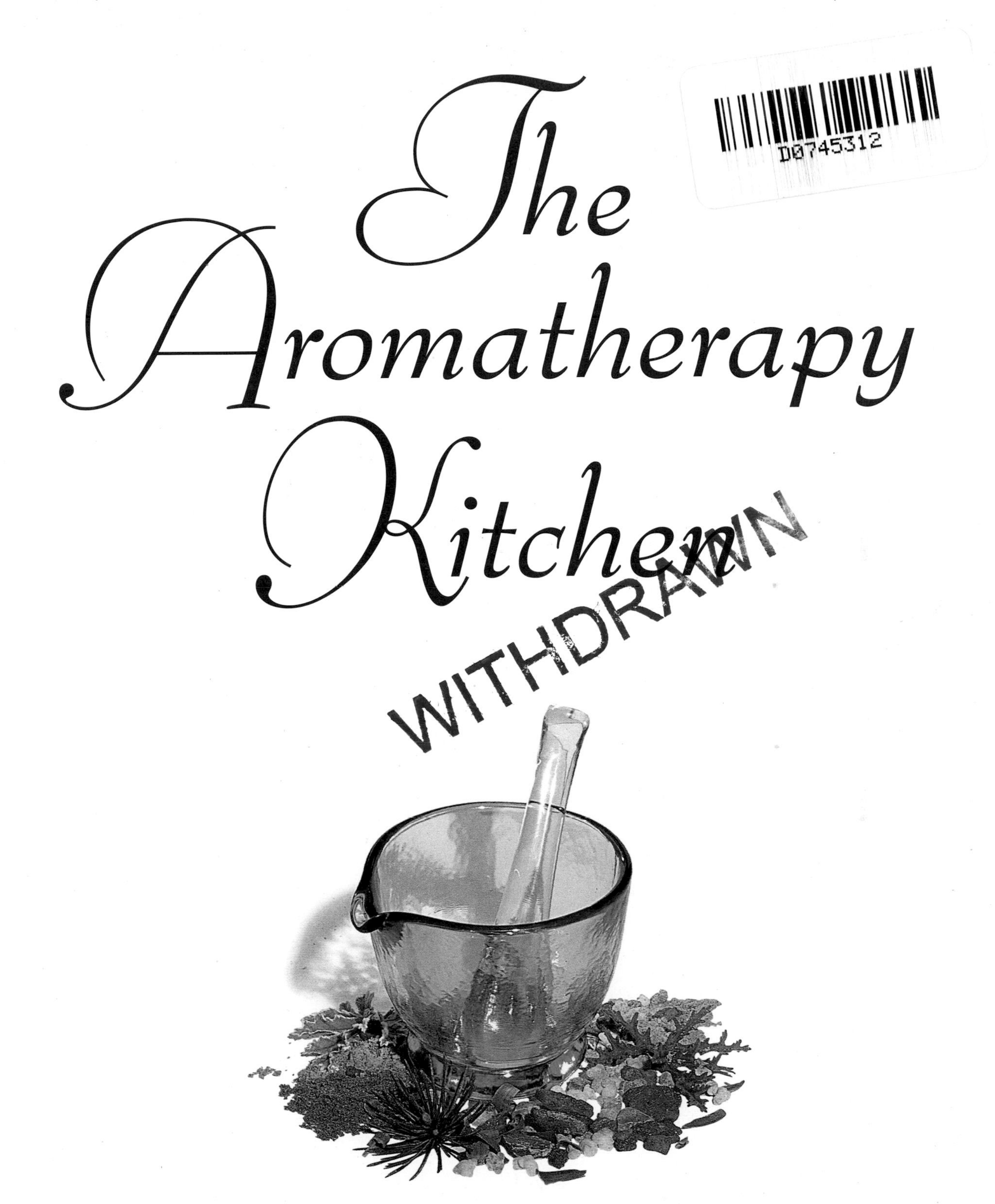

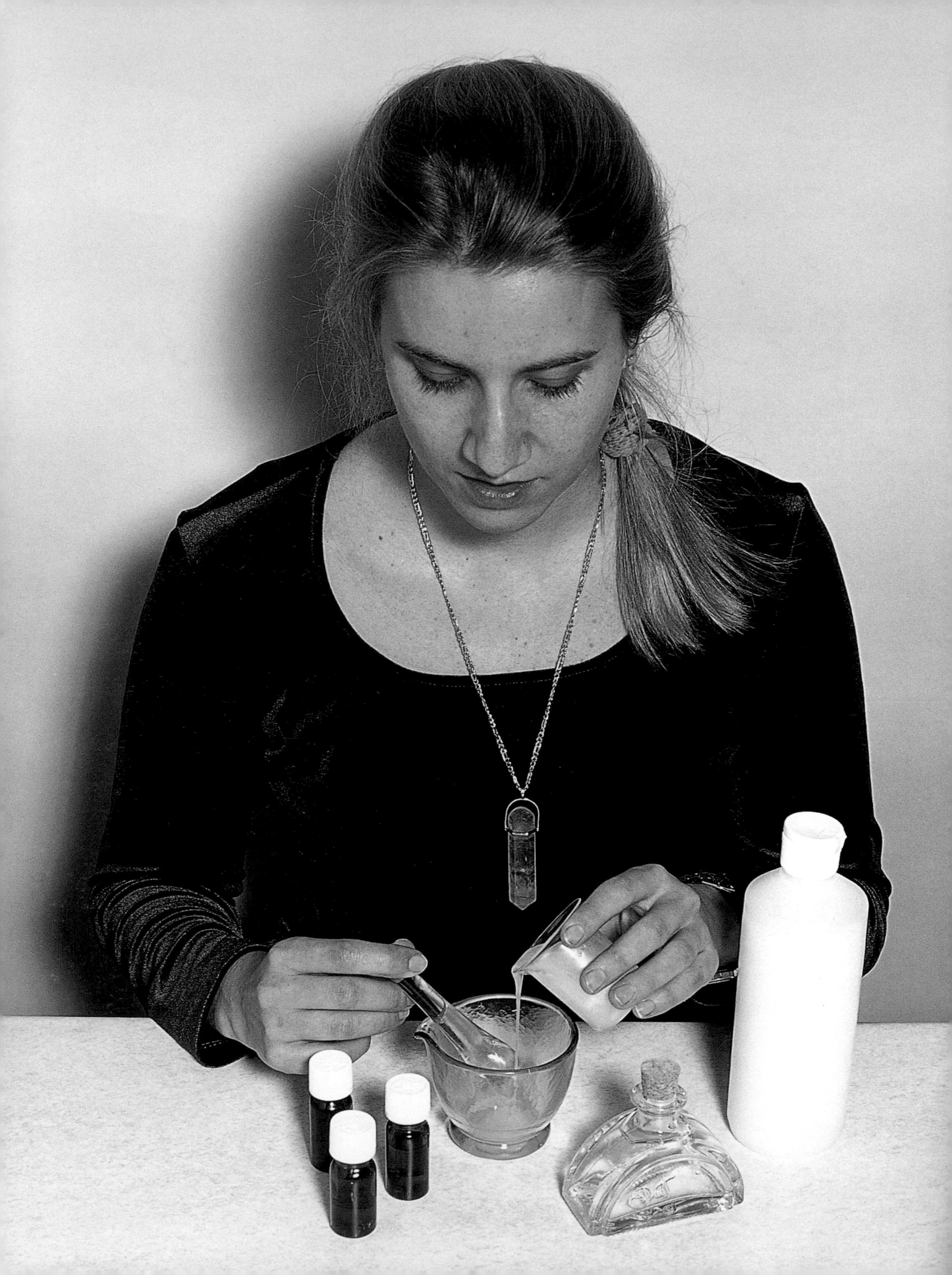

The Aromatherapy Kitchen

Recipes for Health and Beauty using Essential Oils

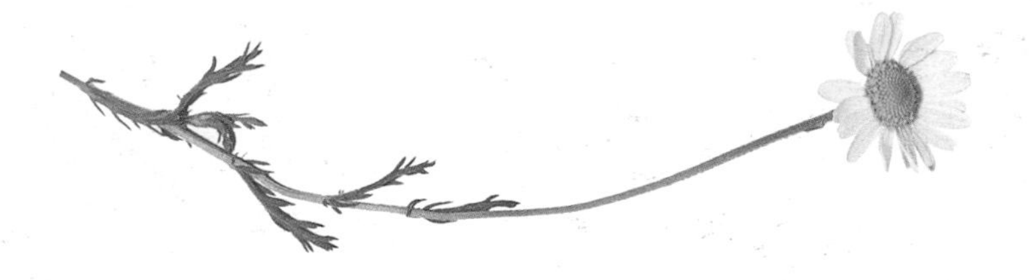

NICOLA JENKINS

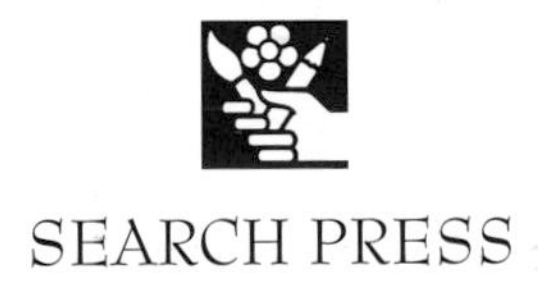

SEARCH PRESS

First published in Great Britain 2001

Search Press Limited
Wellwood, North Farm Road,
Tunbridge Wells, Kent TN2 3DR

ISBN: 0 85532 888 6

Suppliers

If you have difficulty in obtaining any of the materials and equipment mentioned in this book, then please visit the Search Press website for details of suppliers: www.searchpress.com

Alternatively, you can write to the Publishers at the address above, for a current list of stockists, which includes firms who operate a mail-order service.

Publisher's note

All the step-by-step photographs in this book feature the author, Nicola Jenkins, demonstrating how to make natural soaps, creams and cosmetics. No models have been used.

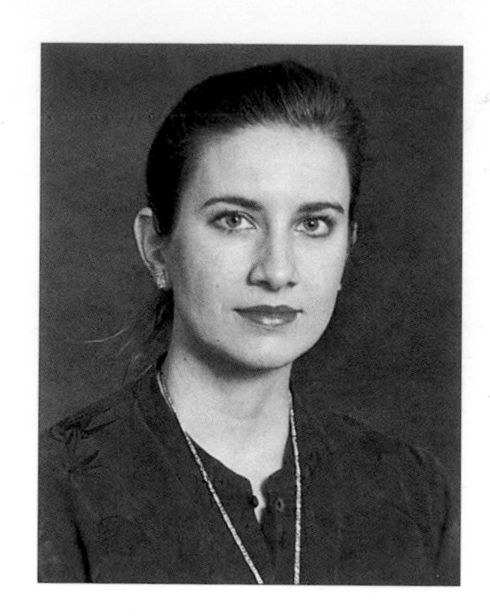

Nicola Jenkins started training as an Aromatherapist while working for a large educational publishing company. Although she never intended for it to be more than a hobby, she later traded in her publishing career to work as a therapist. Several years later, she is now teaching Aromatherapy and Massage in south and west London and practising Aromatherapy and Reflexology in the same areas. Changing the way she worked was, she says, the best decision she ever made – and it all started with a couple of bottles of Lavender and Bergamot essential oils, and a desire to experiment ...

Acknowledgements

A lot of people helped to make this book happen. Thanks to you all, especially to: Diona Gregory, whose encouragement and contacts led me to Search Press and the wonderful experience of working with Roz, Chantal, Lotti, Tamsin and especially Sophie, without whom this might still be gestating; to Robert Tisserand, Jennie Harding and the rest of the staff at the Tisserand Institute, whose Diploma in Holistic Aromatherapy was the most inspiring thing I have ever done; I learnt a huge amount and it has coloured my life ever since. For my family, especially Mum, Tony and Sam, who for some time have been receiving home-made bath products at every opportunity, with no complaints to date. To my friends, clients and ITEC Aromatherapy students, who have also tried all of these recipes in one shape or another.

CONTENTS

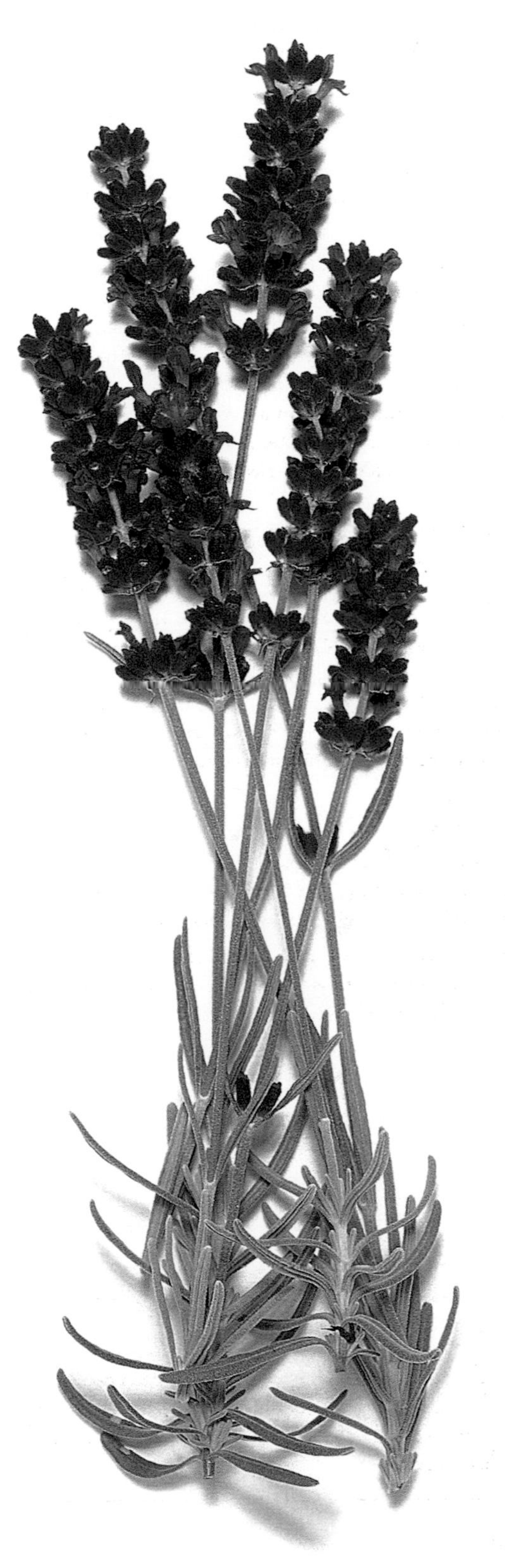

INTRODUCTION

Aromatherapy involves the use of aromatic essential oils which can be inhaled or massaged into the skin to soothe, heal or treat a variety of conditions and ailments. These highly concentrated, beautifully scented oils are extracted from plants and added to carrier oils and base products. As a holistic therapy, aromatherapy works on several levels simultaneously, so helping to relieve conditions affecting the body, mind or spirit, and helping the body to regain its natural balance. So rather than 'curing' ailments, it aims to improve, or maintain, good health. It is not intended to replace medical treatment, but to complement it.

These restorative essential oils have been mentioned throughout history. There is evidence that cave-dwellers used juniper as part of their diet and healthcare; the ancient Egyptians, Persians and Chinese used flower distillations for a variety of conditions and Hippocrates recommended daily massage with scented oils to maintain health and vitality. Today, articles appear regularly in health-related journals referring to the effects essential oils, or blends, can have on us – from treating insomnia in the elderly to encouraging a smooth delivery during labour. Also, it is impossible to visit a pharmacy, or enter a cosmetics department, without seeing essential oil products. Many of these are the result of years of market research, and are excellent if used correctly. However, they lack the personal touch that individual treatments can offer.

You should always take care when buying essential oils, because they may not always be of the highest quality. You need to ensure that they are pure, natural and undiluted, and that they are not being displayed under hot lights, as this may cause them to deteriorate. Better quality oils are available in darkened glass bottles – usually amber or cobalt blue – and these have plastic inserts which allow the liquid to leave the bottles one drop at a time. Unfortunately, the purity of the oils is reflected in the price. The more difficult it is to extract them from the plants, the more expensive they become. Prices also vary according to the weather; they may rise if there has been a poor crop during the year.

Most essential oils will last for approximately two years before they start to degrade, then their fragrance will start to fade or develop oily, rancid undertones. Citrus oils such as Grapefruit, Bergamot, Lemon, Orange, Mandarin and Lime will last only six months before this begins to happen. You can extend their shelf life if you store them in a cool, dark place. The ideal location is the fridge. If you store them here you may want to invest in an airtight container with a lid, so that their scent does not mingle with the food. Failing this, keep them stored in dark glass jars and in a box, away from children, sunlight and any sudden temperature changes.

Professional Aromatherapists offer treatments at recognised centres or clinics, but if you want to use essential oils at home and do not know where to start, I will show you how. This book is not about aromatherapy massage. It shows instead how essential oils can be used to help many minor conditions, looking at simple, quick, inexpensive ways of creating shampoos, creams, cleansers, toners, perfumes – and more. I have included a selection of oils, some of the conditions they can treat and many different recipes. Basic information is given on how they can be mixed and matched with existing readily available products, and clear step-by-step photographs illustrate how to blend them safely.

Finally, I hope you enjoy using the recipes in this book, and that in doing so you discover the pleasure of learning about the wonderful qualities of essential oils.

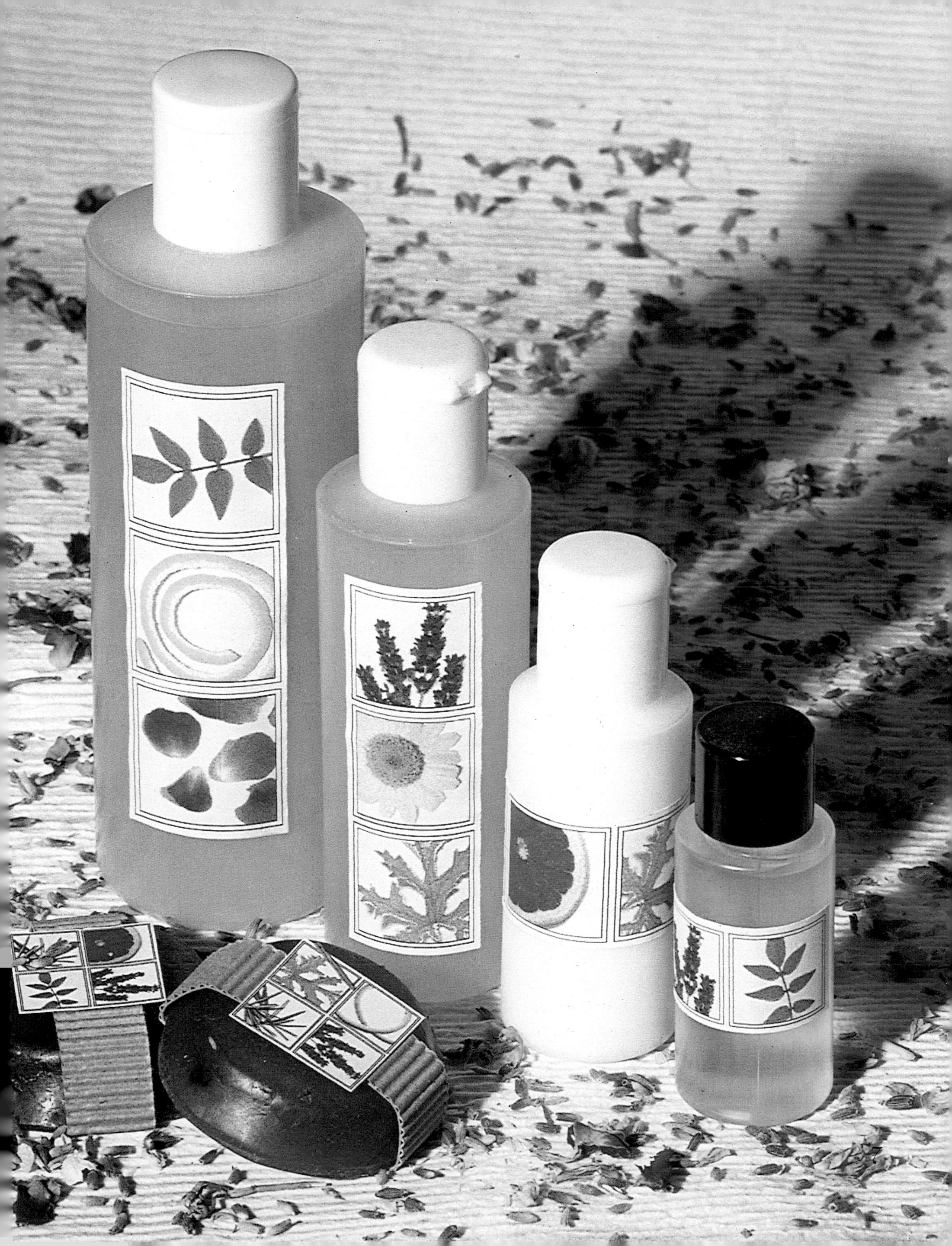

Essential Oils

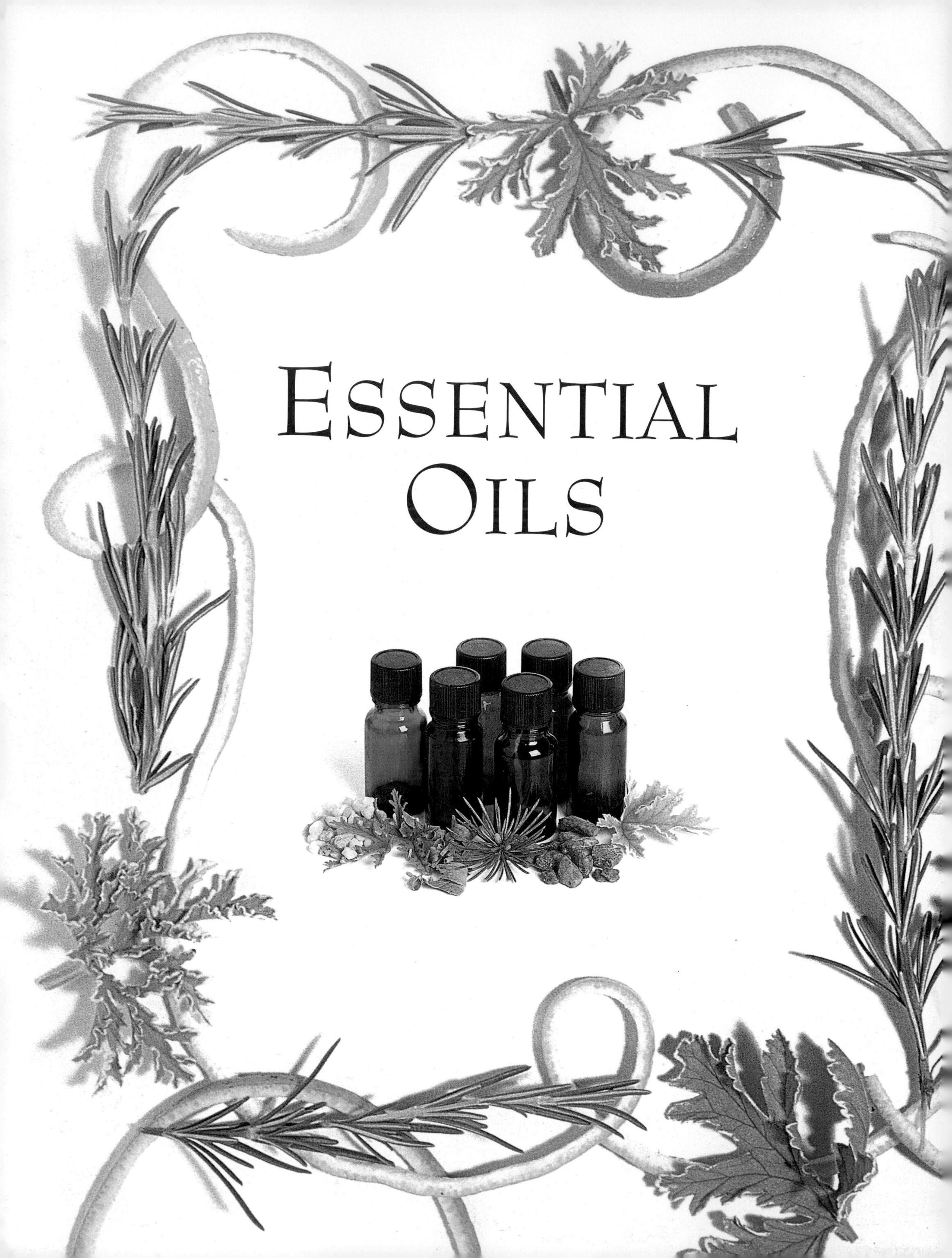

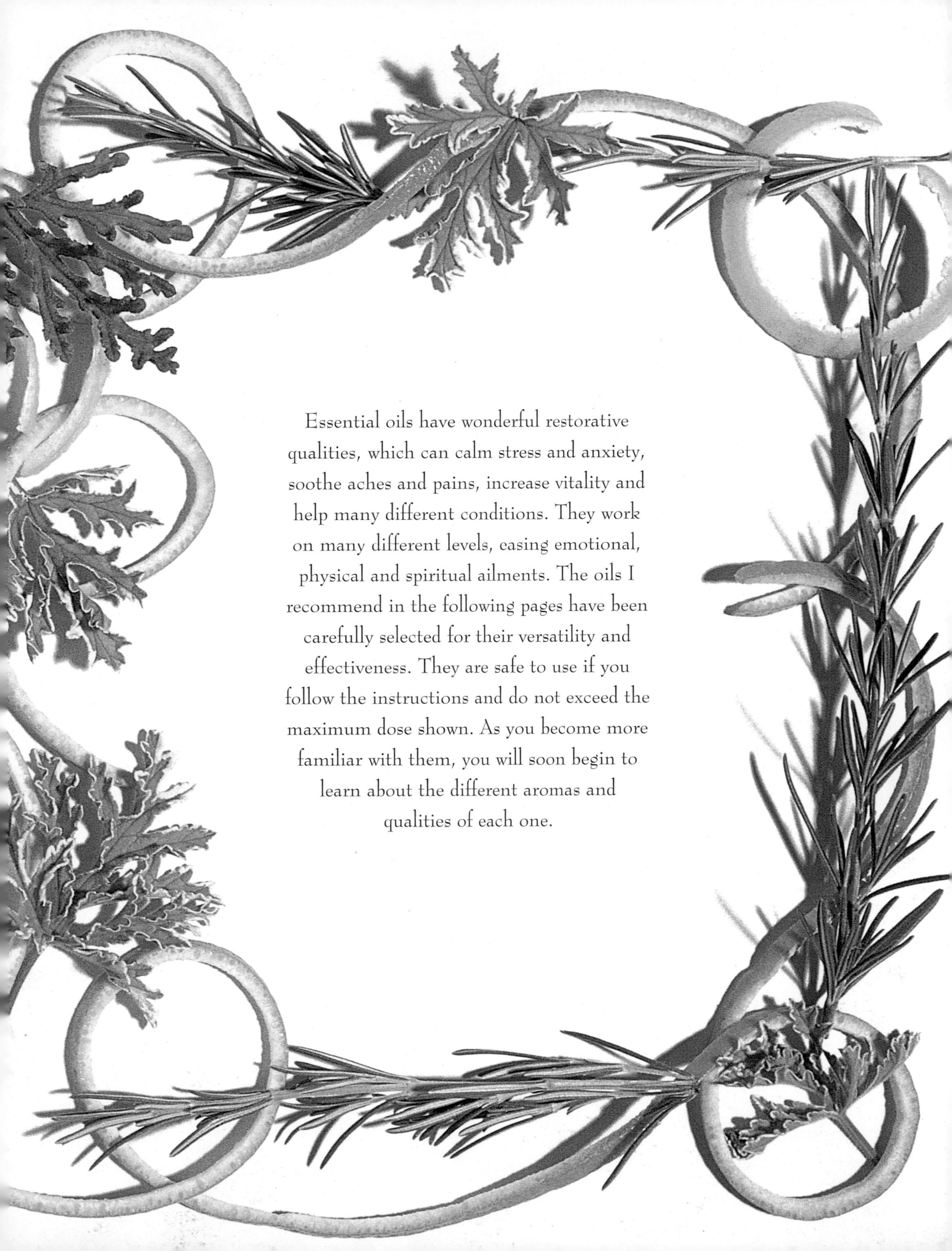

Essential oils have wonderful restorative qualities, which can calm stress and anxiety, soothe aches and pains, increase vitality and help many different conditions. They work on many different levels, easing emotional, physical and spiritual ailments. The oils I recommend in the following pages have been carefully selected for their versatility and effectiveness. They are safe to use if you follow the instructions and do not exceed the maximum dose shown. As you become more familiar with them, you will soon begin to learn about the different aromas and qualities of each one.

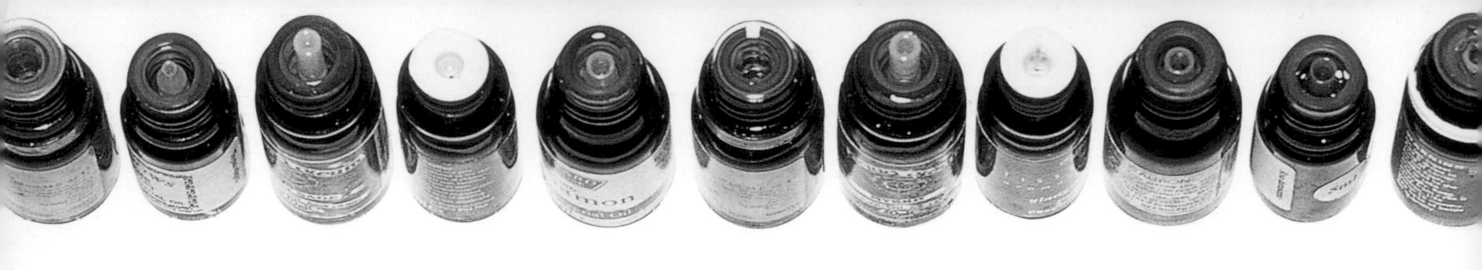

Health & Safety

When choosing your oil from the Index by Symptom (see pages 62–63), you will notice that a number of them can be used to treat the same condition or different conditions. I have offered suggestions throughout the book which will help you make the right choice. Essential oils are powerful chemicals, with wonderful therapeutic qualities. If you follow the advice in this section, you should benefit from these qualities without experiencing any adverse effects.

- Keep essential oils out of reach of children.
- Never apply essential oils to open wounds.
- Always check that you are not allergic to the essential oil or the carrier oil you have chosen, by using the patch test explained below.
- If you suffer an adverse reaction to any products containing essential oils, contact your doctor immediately.
- Check with an Aromatherapist before applying essential oils to damaged skin.
- Some oils increase sensitivity to sunlight or ultraviolet light, so always check with an Aromatherapist before using them.
- Never digest essential oils. They should only be applied to the skin or inhaled.
- Essential oils must always be diluted with carrier oils or a base product.
- If you accidentally splash neat essential oil on your skin, wash the area quickly, then apply unperfumed lotion.
- Keep essential oils away from your eyes. If you get diluted essential oil in your eyes, wash them out immediately with clean, warm water. If you get neat oil in your eyes, immediately flush out with cold full fat milk. If this does not relieve the stinging, consult your doctor.
- The oils in this book have been chosen carefully, as there is no toxicity risk providing you follow all the dosage instructions. For advice on using other essential oils, contact a qualified Aromatherapist.

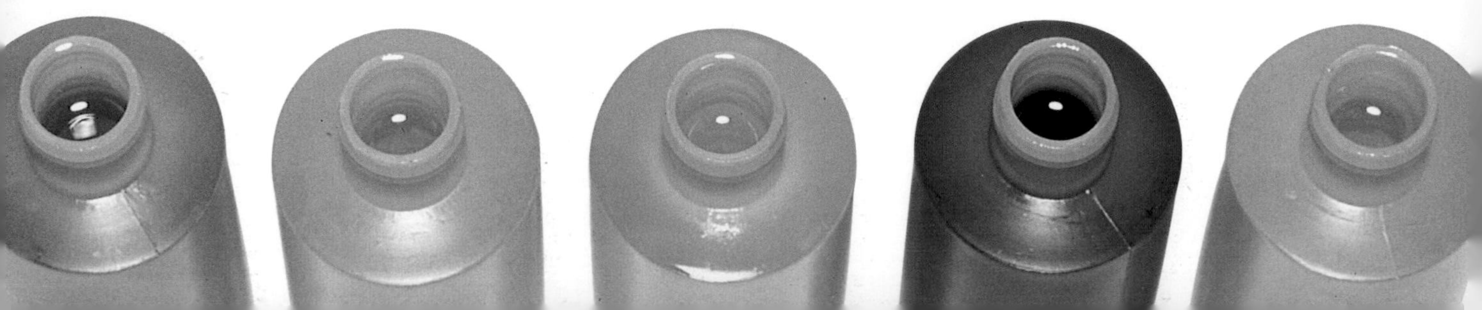

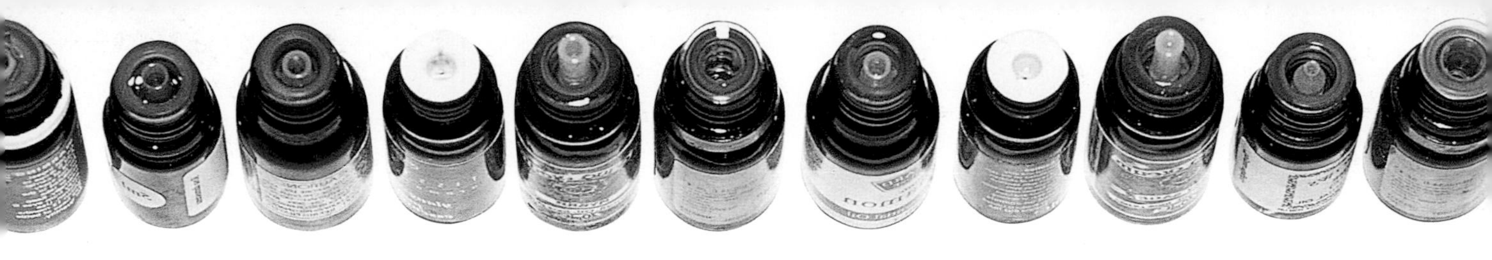

Allergies

If you suffer from food allergies, the related essential oils must not be used. For example, avoid Lemon, Bergamot, Orange and Grapefruit oils if you react to citrus fruit; they are extracted from the fruit peel, which contains substances to which some allergy sufferers might react. Neroli and Petitgrain are extracted from the flowers and leaves. A reaction to these oils is unlikely, but allergy sufferers should carry out the patch test before use.

Wheat allergy sufferers should avoid Wheatgerm oil as a carrier, and nut allergy sufferers should not choose Avocado, Peanut and Sweet Almond oils. Please note that there are plenty of other carrier oils which can be used by allergy sufferers with no risk of reaction – try Jojoba, Grapeseed or Peach Kernel.

If you have experienced allergic reactions before, do a patch test before using an oil for the first time. If you have no specific allergies but have a very sensitive skin, limit the amount you use to less than half the recommended dose for an adult. Also, note that Lemongrass, Jasmine and Rosemary can cause a reaction, so are best avoided. If you are particularly keen to use them, carry out a patch test first.

If you do have a reaction to one of the products, immediately wash the affected area with clean water. Alternatively, a cream containing 8 drops of Lavender in 20g (0.7oz) of moisturiser, or a spray containing a drop of Lavender in 30ml (1fl oz) of water, in a mister, will help calm the reaction.

Epilepsy

Avoid Rosemary. All other essential oils mentioned in this book can be used as for a healthy adult.

High blood pressure

Of the essential oils mentioned in this book, Rosemary and Peppermint are the only ones that need to be avoided by those who suffer from high blood pressure.

Fevers

It is best to avoid using Rosemary or Peppermint if you have a fever. Essential oils of particular use in reducing fevers include Lavender, Lemongrass, Palmarosa, Lemon and Bergamot.

Homeopathic remedies

If you are receiving homeopathic treatment, you should consult your homoeopath before using essential oils. Some, such as Rosemary, Peppermint, Eucalyptus, Tea Tree, Manuka, Cinnamon, Bay and Clove, can interfere with prescribed remedies.

Patch test

Put 2 drops of the oil on to a plaster, then stick the plaster to the inside of your forearm. If you are allergic to plasters, use gauze held in place by hypoallergenic adhesive strips. Leave it in place for 24 hours. If you experience no reaction in that time, it is safe to proceed with care.

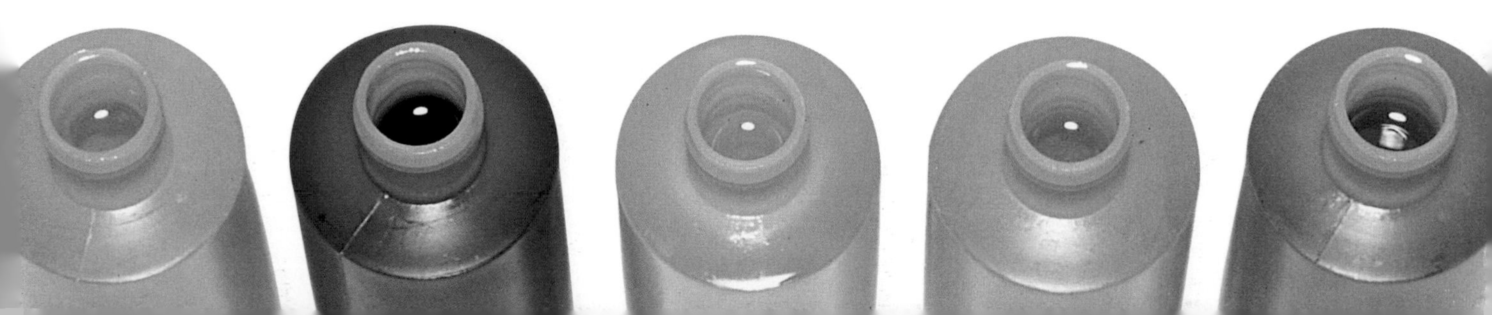

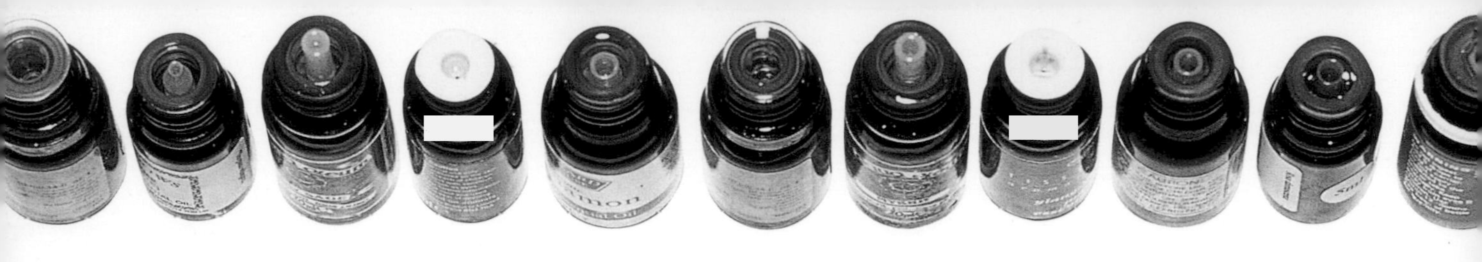

Pregnancy and breast-feeding

Aromatherapists advise that it is best to stay away from most essential oils while you are pregnant, especially in the first trimester, if you are having a difficult pregnancy, or if you have any history of miscarriage.

However, massage can be extremely beneficial to a pregnant woman. As well as helping to ease backache, it can reduce water retention, improve circulation, encourage restful sleep and reduce some of the side effects of pregnancy – nausea, painful breasts and sudden mood swings.

Luckily, a few oils are considered completely safe during the later stages of a normal pregnancy, and if you stick to these, you should be able to enjoy all the benefits of an Aromatherapy massage just when you need them most! After the first trimester, and if you have no history of miscarriage, it is safe to use Neroli, Lavender and both Chamomiles. Geranium, Patchouli, Petitgrain and Sandalwood can be used in small doses for calming and uplifting purposes. In the last trimester you can add Rose to this list, at which point it becomes extremely useful in preparing the body for labour.

During pregnancy the skin is slightly more sensitive, the sense of smell is a lot stronger and if used, the majority of essential oils will also be experienced by the foetus. You should therefore halve the recommended healthy adult dose. If you are in any doubt at all, you should consult an experienced Aromatherapist.

Avoid Rosemary and Tea Tree when breast-feeding. If you are having trouble breast-feeding, creams containing Jasmine, Lemongrass, Geranium, Roman Chamomile, Lavender or Peppermint can help to ease some of the symptoms.

Learning about the oils

You should familiarise yourself with the oils before you start using them. Their aromas change over time and they also change when they are blended together, so you will need to try this simple test.

Place one drop of a single essential oil on a tissue or cotton bud, then smell it immediately – this first scent is described as the top note.

Wait for two minutes, then smell the oil again. This is the middle note. Ask yourself whether the aroma has changed. How do you feel about it now?

Wait for another six minutes, then smell the oil once more. This is the base note. Has it changed again? It probably has.

Dosage

The essential oils used in this book must be diluted in a carrier oil or other base product. They should not be used in their pure form. In the following pages I recommend the dosages, talk about the plants and flowers, and show you the best way to blend your own shampoos, bath products, soaps, creams, oils and perfumes.

Healthy adults

The recommendation for healthy adults is a maximum of 2% of essential oils in any carrier solution, whether it be a vegetable oil or a base product such as shower gel, shampoo, bubble bath or moisturiser. This would be 8 drops in total in 20ml (0.6fl oz) of a liquid carrier product. For example, if you are using three essential oils in a recipe, the total amount should be 8 drops in 20ml (0.6fl oz).

With creams, use 2% of essential oils. This would be 20 drops in 50g (1.8oz) of moisturiser or

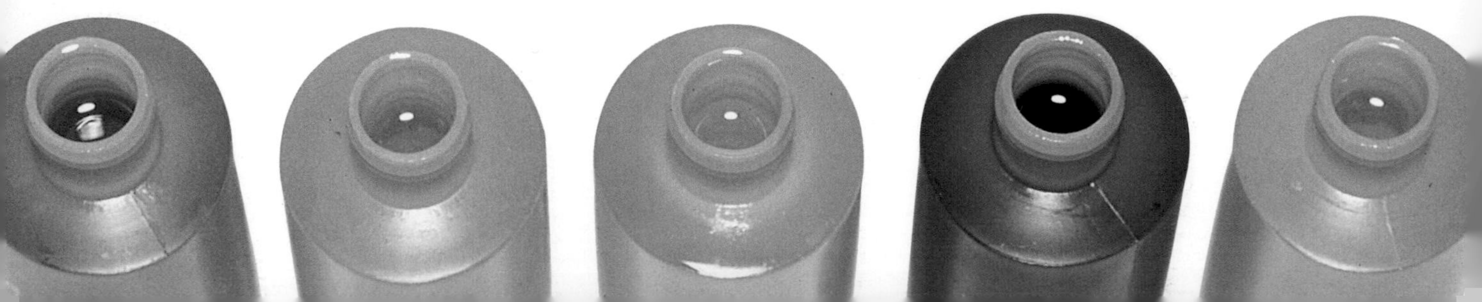

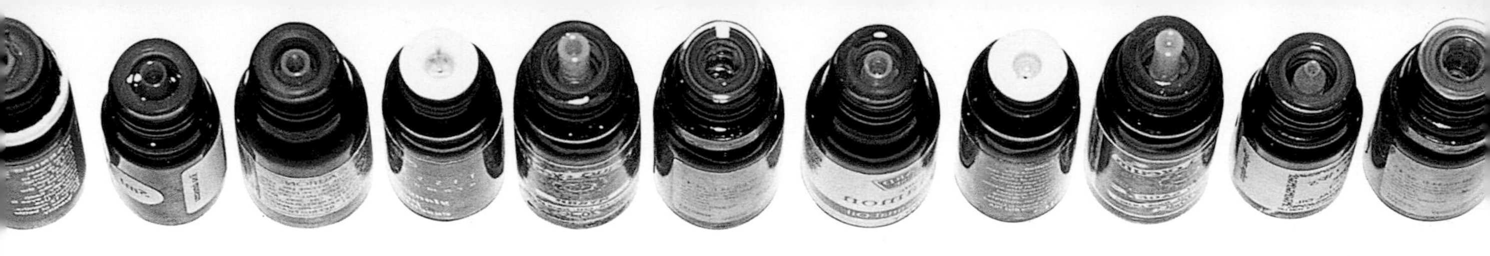

any similar, non-liquid base. Halve the dosage if you are using a cream on cracked, raw or sensitive skin.

When making soap, the essential oil dosage can be raised to 3%, which allows for evaporation during the soap making process. This is 35 drops per 50g (1.8oz) of the hard soap used as a base.

If an extra drop should accidentally fall into the remedy, add more carrier oil or base product to dilute the solution to a safe level.

Infants

Infants under two years of age have sensitive and relatively porous skin, so only 2 drops of essential oil should be used in 100ml (3.2fl oz) of carrier oil or base product. Lavender, Roman Chamomile and Orange are particularly effective in helping infants to sleep soundly, at easing nightmares, keeping colds at bay and in treating minor skin conditions such as cradle cap and nappy rash. Other oils, particularly Rosemary, Lemongrass, Jasmine or Eucalyptus, should be treated with great care, because an infant's skin is so sensitive. Vaporisers placed in the child's room are a harmless and effective method of encouraging sleep or soothing coughs and colds. One drop each of Roman Chamomile, Benzoin and Orange in a vaporiser are particularly effective for children experiencing nightmares.

Children under twelve

All essential oils are safe for children, providing you halve the adult dose (see page 12). Children under twelve are prone to cuts, scrapes and insect bites and stings – all of which can be helped by essential oils like Lavender, Roman Chamomile or Lemon. As adults, we can also underestimate the amount of stress children face, whether from peer pressure, bullying or feeling insecure and under-appreciated. Benzoin, Neroli, Vetiver, Peppermint and Patchouli are all very useful in helping them to feel more confident, easing nightmares and stopping butterflies wreaking havoc in small stomachs.

Carrier oils

Most essential oils must not be used undiluted if you are applying them to your skin, so a carrier oil should be used. This literally 'carries' the essential oils, diluting them to a safe level. Essential oils dissolve most readily in vegetable oils, all of which are excellent carriers. They are also rich in vitamins and therefore nourish the skin as well.

Some of the more popular carrier oils include Grapeseed, Jojoba, Hazelnut, Avocado, Calendula, Sunflower Seed, Macadamia Nut, Sweet Almond and Peach Kernel, and they all have slightly different properties. Whilst Grapeseed, Sweet Almond and Peach Kernel are probably most commonly used for massage oils, others can be used to help certain ailments or conditions. Calendula, for example, encourages stretch marks to fade and helps reduce scar tissue. Jojoba oil, when used as a face oil, can help to maintain more mature skin, and it helps to reduce fine lines. It also dissolves sebum, the skin's naturally occurring oil, so it is excellent for removing dirt from the pores. Avocado oil is absorbed into drier, finer facial skin quickly, and it makes an excellent moisturiser.

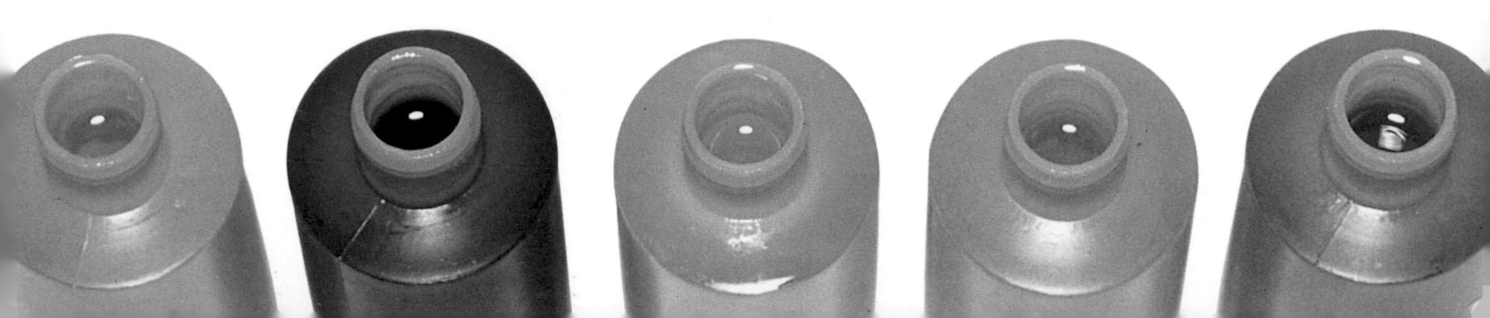

Flowers

Flowers are the reproductive organs of plants. It is interesting therefore to note that many of the flowering plant essential oils can reduce discomforts associated with reproductive system disorders. There is usually a flower that will help restore the body's natural balance, whether you are suffering from painful periods, pre-menstrual tension, menopausal symptoms, infertility, lack of sexual appetite, prostatitis or the effects of pregnancy and childbirth (see the Health and Safety section on pregnancy). However, there are many more reasons for using these essential oils.

Chamomile

Matricaria chamomilla or *Anthemis nobilis*

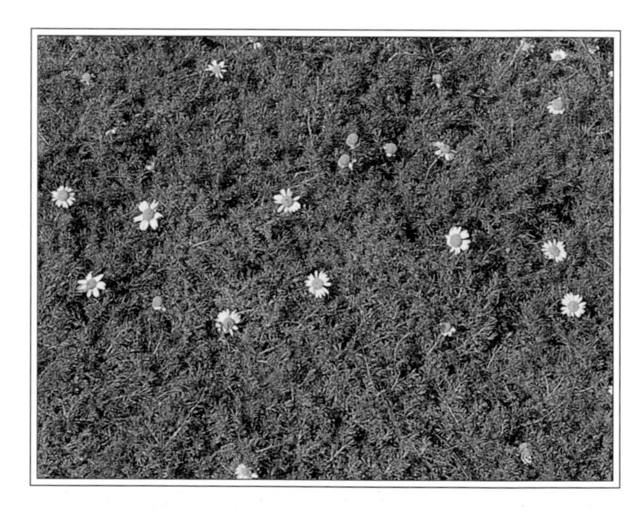

There are several different kinds of chamomile. *Matricaria chamomilla* (German Chamomile) and *Anthemis nobilis* (Roman Chamomile) are just two. German Chamomile is recognised by its deep blue colour. However, not everyone likes its strong, herbaceous aroma. If you mix it with the lighter and sweeter oils, it slides gently into the background, giving the blend a hidden strength. You will never need to use large amounts, so buy the smallest quantity you can find. If you do not like it, try Roman Chamomile instead – it does not have the distinctive colour of the German Chamomile but it is sweeter, with an apple-like aroma and the same qualities.

Chamomile is an extremely good anti-inflammatory essential oil, which makes it wonderfully soothing for most forms of arthritis and muscular aches and pains – especially where there is some swelling. It is also good for neuralgia, painful periods, irritable bowel syndrome, eczema and burns. It is a strong sedative and useful if you suffer from long-standing insomnia or tension. Both Chamomiles can be used safely during the later stages of a normal pregnancy.

Maximum dose *2 drops in 20ml (0.6fl oz) carrier oil*

Geranium

Pelargonium graveolens

This favourite summer flowering plant, loved for its interesting foliage and bright, colourful blossoms, can be seen decorating balconies and windowsills all over Europe. The essential oil is distilled from the leaves of the plant, and some of the chemicals that are present are the same as those contained in the more expensive Rose oil. Geranium oil is often used instead of Rose oil, so if you are offered an inexpensive Rose, be careful – you may be buying the wrong oil.

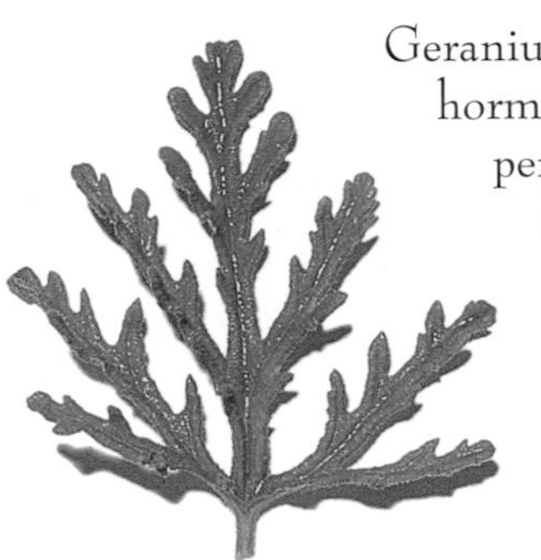

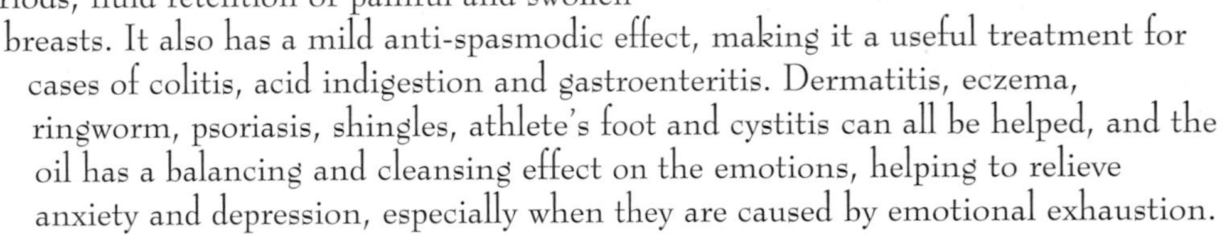

Geranium oil is extremely effective for regulating hormonal imbalances, which appear as painful periods, fluid retention or painful and swollen breasts. It also has a mild anti-spasmodic effect, making it a useful treatment for cases of colitis, acid indigestion and gastroenteritis. Dermatitis, eczema, ringworm, psoriasis, shingles, athlete's foot and cystitis can all be helped, and the oil has a balancing and cleansing effect on the emotions, helping to relieve anxiety and depression, especially when they are caused by emotional exhaustion.

Maximum dose *3 drops in 20ml (0.6fl oz) carrier oil*

Jasmine

Jasminum officianale

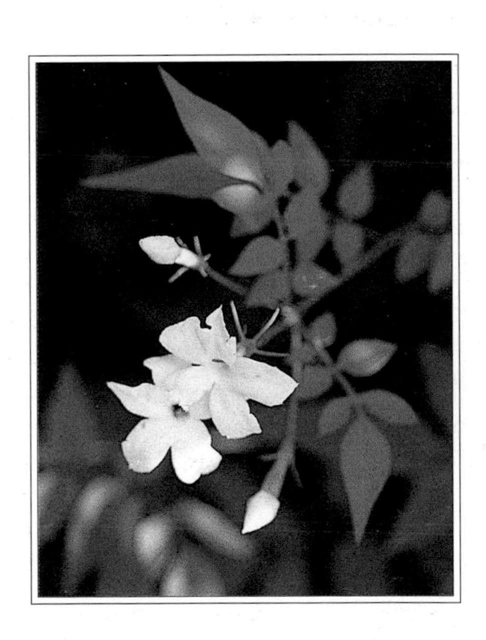

Sometimes called 'Queen of the Night', Jasmine accounts for the rich heady note which graces so many of the floral perfumes available today. Perhaps part of the reason it appears in so many perfumes is because it is thought to be an aphrodisiac. It is closely associated with reproductive functions, and is an effective relief for painful periods and PMS. It helps to improve appetites for life and intimacy too – in both men and women.

If you are prone to allergic reactions, do a patch test first (see page 11). Jasmine can irritate sensitive skins.

Maximum dose *2 drops in 20ml (0.6fl oz) carrier oil*

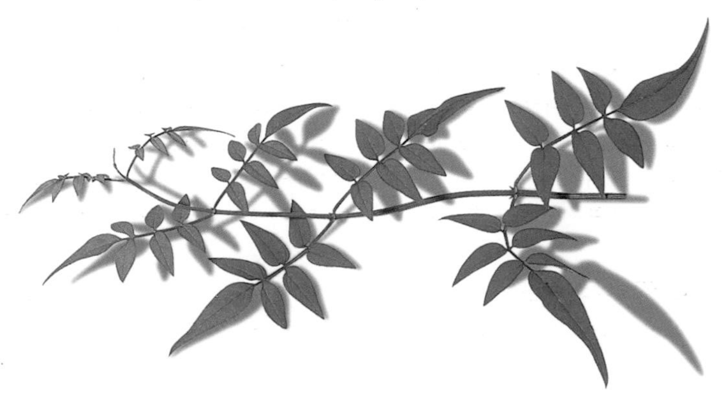

Lavender

Lavandula angustifolia

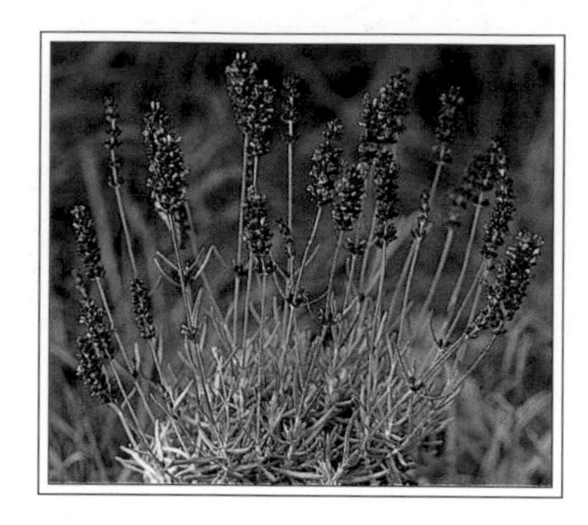

Lavender is non-toxic, adaptable and it can be used for just about anything – even serious conditions. It can be used during the later stages of a normal pregnancy and on infants, and even undiluted on scalds – and if applied quickly it will prevent blistering. It calms eczema, dermatitis, acne and boils, and soothes muscular aches, insect bites and stings. As a gentle sedative it is very effective, helping to relieve insomnia, stress, anxiety and depression, and it helps to lower blood pressure, reduce headaches and migraines, ease nausea, constipation, thrush and cystitis. It can also be helpful in treating athlete's foot, scabies, lice and intestinal parasites.

Maximum dose *4 drops in 20ml (0.6fl oz) carrier oil*

Neroli

Citrus aurantium

Tradition has it that Neroli, or Orange Blossom, was used in the floral headdresses of many a shy or unwilling bride. Aromatherapists still use it today for people who have experienced severe shock, extreme anxiety or great levels of stress. This is a wonderful but expensive essential oil to have to hand if someone you know is facing exams, interviews or life-changing events. In times of crisis you may not have time to make a cream or lotion for them – in which case, just get them to inhale a couple of drops of Neroli on a tissue. It really can make a difference. Neroli helps to quieten the heart when it is pounding with fear, it calms butterflies and soothes nervous indigestion and diarrhoea. It can be used safely in the later stages of a normal pregnancy. It is also beneficial in rejuvenating mature skin and preventing stretch marks if used regularly.

Maximum dose *3 drops in 20ml (0.6fl oz) carrier oil*

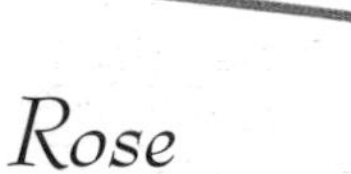

Rose

Rosa centifolia or *Rosa damascena*

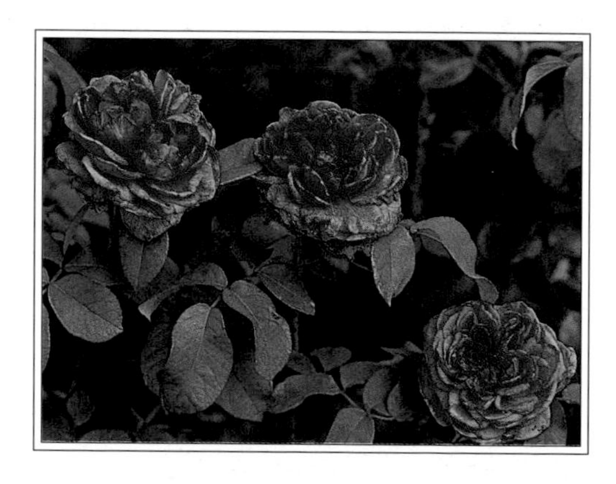

There are two forms of essential oil: *Rosa centifolia* (Rose Absolute) and *Rosa damascena* (Rose Otto), and they are each extracted by different methods. Either can be used, but you might want to try the Rose Absolute first. It has a distinctive red colour, and some people feel that it smells of garden roses during the summer, whereas Rose Otto has a slightly sharper, more medicinal smell. The latter is often better used for physical conditions such as painful periods, dry skin or addictions.

Rose is extremely useful for menopausal symptoms like hot flushes, insomnia and emotional swings. It is closely associated with the skin and can help to heal cracked or dry skin, rejuvenate mature skin, and soothe scars and thread veins. It can also be used to dispel feelings of anger, fear, disappointment, grief, irritability and resentment, and I have seen it used effectively to support those recovering from various addictive states. It helps to calm nerves and dispel the anxieties that are associated with cravings. It can be used safely in the last trimester of pregnancy, when it helps prepare the body for labour.

Maximum dose *1 drop in 20ml (0.6fl oz) carrier oil*

Resins

Resins or gums are the sap of the tree. If you think of amber, that slowly leaking resin which has preserved insects and plant life for thousands of years, you will see why the oils can be used to help heal wounds, relieve aches and pains, rejuvenate the skin and support the immune system. They also ease breathing difficulties.

Benzoin

Stryax benzoin

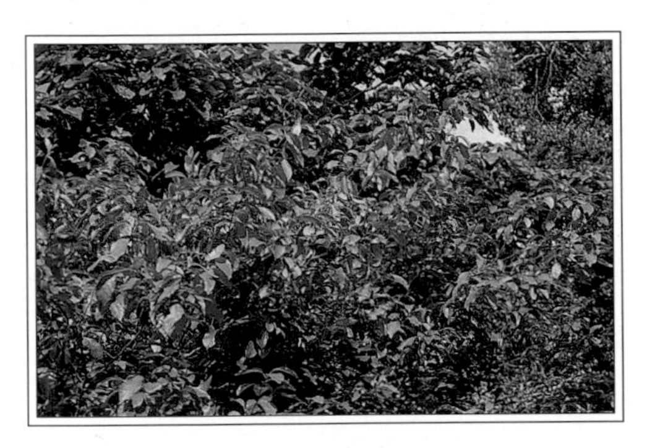

Benzoin has been used in Europe since the fourteenth century, despite the fact that its origins lie in the islands of the South Pacific. It is one of the main ingredients of 'Friar's Balsam' – the other ingredient is Frankincense. 'Friar's Balsam' is used extensively for cracked skin and chest infections and Benzoin is a particularly effective remedy for both these conditions. Its vanilla-like scent gives it a sweet note, which makes having a chesty cough, catarrh, bronchitis, psoriasis, sinusitis or impetigo less unpleasant, and it makes a nice change from the medicinal essential oils more frequently used as inhalants for chest conditions. Benzoin is also very useful in aiding insomnia, anxiety and panic attacks.

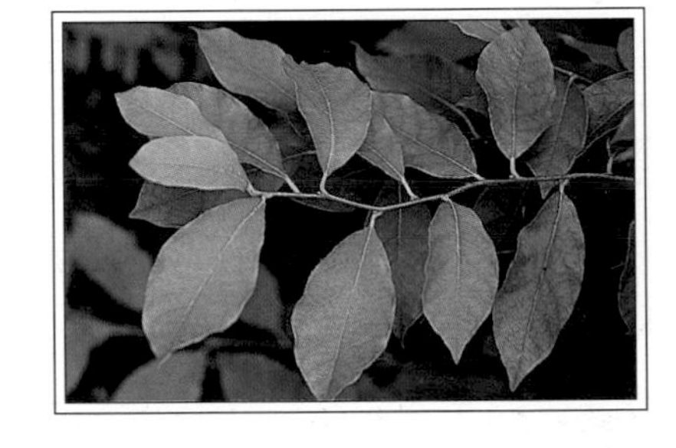

Maximum dose *2 drops in 20ml (0.6fl oz) carrier oil*

Frankincense

Boswellia carterii

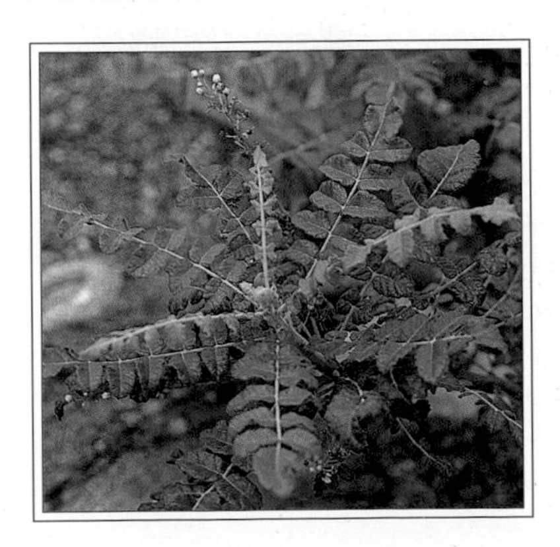

Frankincense is one of the essential oils for which there is early documentary evidence of its use – both for medicinal, and for meditative purposes. The ancient Egyptians used it as part of the embalming process, and the Bible refers to it as one of the gifts presented to Jesus at his birth.

Frankincense is extremely good for relieving muscular aches and pains and clearing chest conditions – coughs, colds, catarrh and laryngitis. It helps to fortify the mind and to encourage deep breathing. It has been used throughout history in places of worship, as it encourages a meditative state of mind, while being uplifting and comforting.

Maximum dose *3 drops in 20ml (0.6fl oz) carrier oil*

Wood

Extracting essential oils from wood is a difficult task. It usually involves a great deal of time, as wood and bark are not the easiest of substances to distil. Although these essential oils are effective, the oils of some trees are so sought after that the demand is often reflected in the price. Rosewood, for example, is so highly prized that the search for this oil is said to have contributed, in some part, to the deforestation of the Brazilian rainforests. Many Aromatherapists are now turning to Japanese Ho Wood as a rainforest-friendly alternative. Sandalwood, from Mysore in India, is also in such demand that its export is severely limited and adulteration is rife. These oils are wonderful for improving skin conditions and are also closely linked with respiration and the immune system. Think of them as oils that can give you the strength of a tree – to grow tall and healthy in the sun.

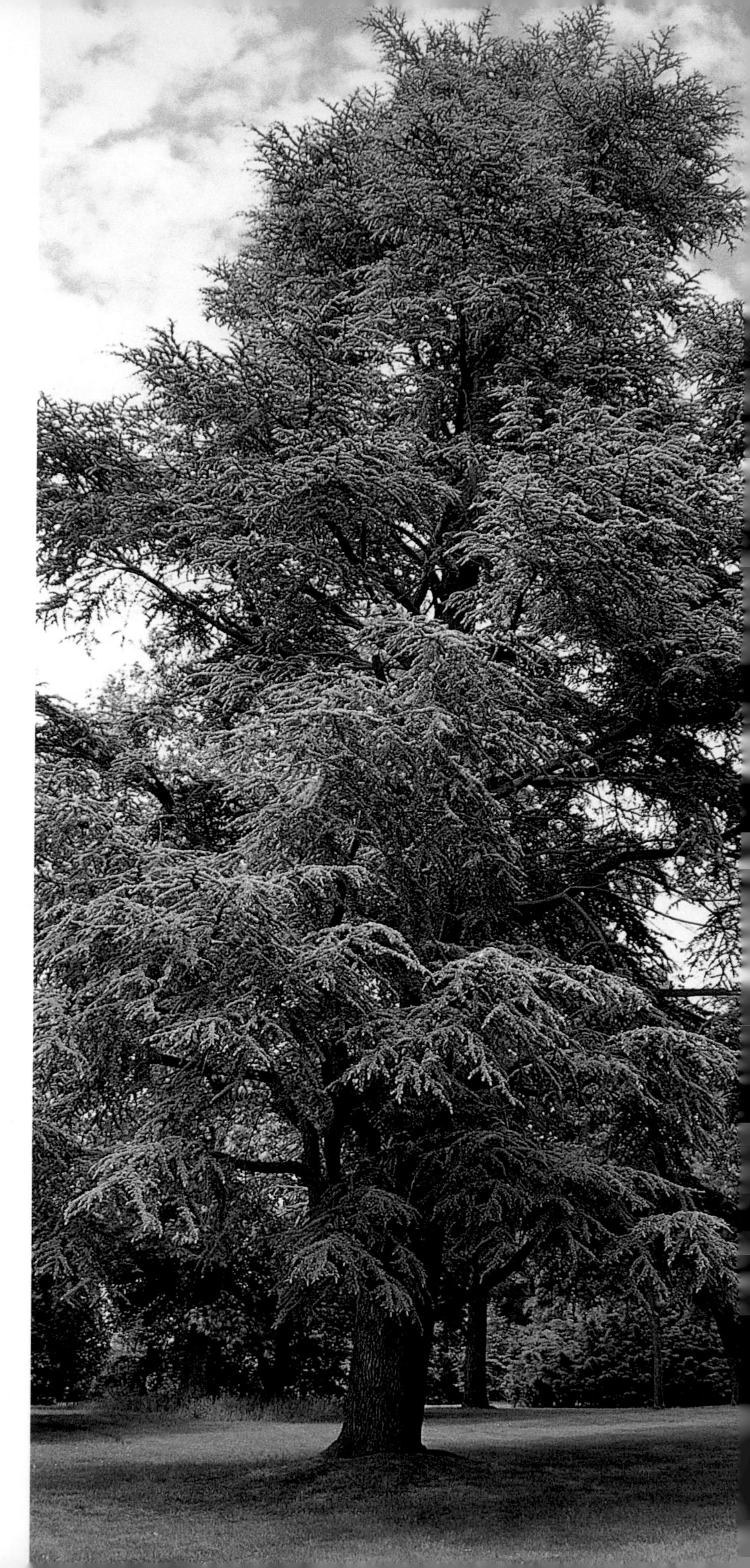

Cedarwood

Cedrus atlantica or *Juniperus virginiana*

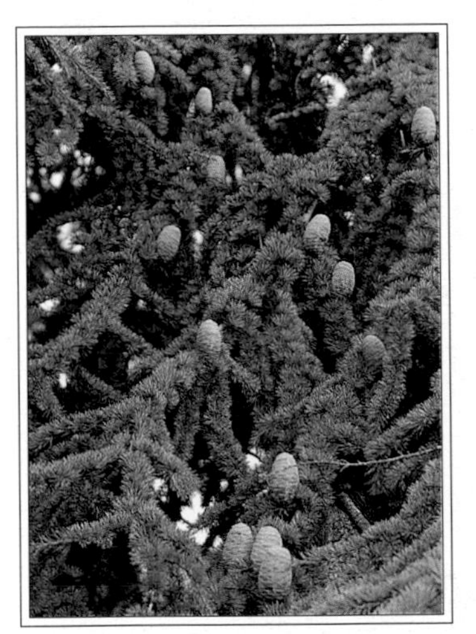

There are two main types of Cedarwood essential oils. They are made from *Cedrus atlantica (*Atlas Cedar) and *Juniperus virginiana* (Virginian or Texan Cedar). I would recommend Atlas Cedar because it has a gentler, softer and sweeter note, and because it is extremely good for a variety of skin conditions. Virginian Cedar is more astringent, with a sharper, more herbaceous note. Both oils are extremely good for clearing acne and they can also ease the breathing of asthma sufferers. Weeping and dry eczema will see a real improvement if

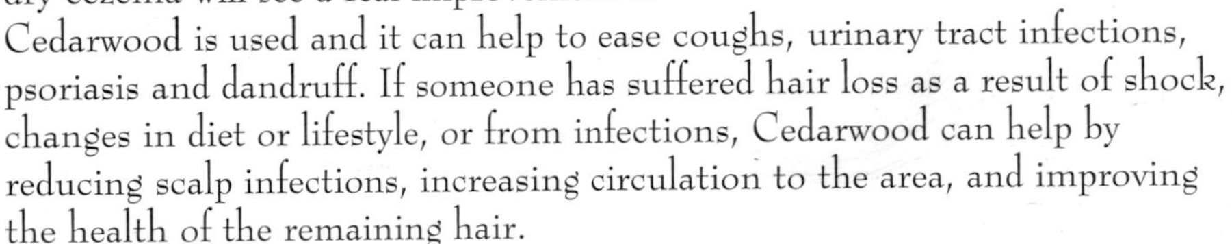

Cedarwood is used and it can help to ease coughs, urinary tract infections, psoriasis and dandruff. If someone has suffered hair loss as a result of shock, changes in diet or lifestyle, or from infections, Cedarwood can help by reducing scalp infections, increasing circulation to the area, and improving the health of the remaining hair.

Maximum dose *2 drops in 20ml (0.6fl oz) carrier oil*

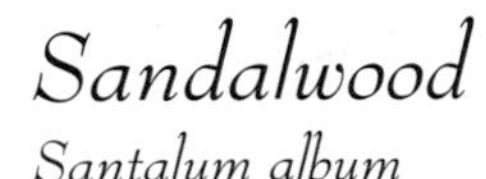

Sandalwood

Santalum album

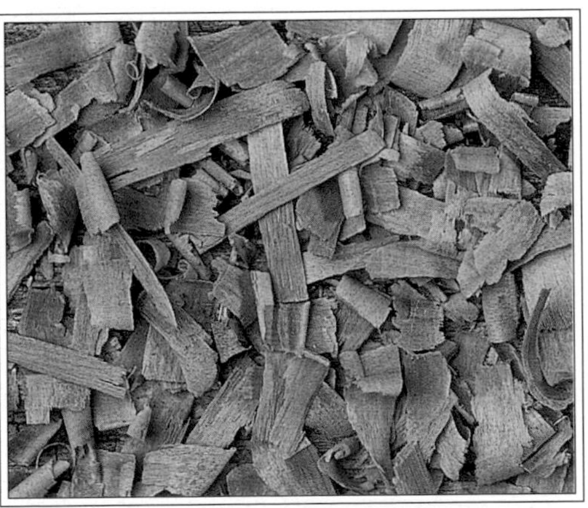

Sandalwood is found in many male cosmetics. It has a dry, musky odour which is sedating, and has the reputation of being a mild aphrodisiac. It is effective for clearing acne and balancing either oily or dry skin, and it is also good for reducing the pain of cystitis. It is an expectorant and will help clear phlegm from mucusy coughs or chronic bronchitis. It is also extremely useful for sore throats – if you smooth your chosen blend on your neck, you will immediately feel relief. Sandalwood renews feelings of self-confidence and power, and its link with sore throats may explain why it is also good at easing the frustration some people feel when they have difficulty expressing themselves.

Maximum dose *4 drops in 20ml (0.6fl oz) carrier oil*

Rosewood

Aniba rosaeodora

Rosewood is a main ingredient in many cosmetics, and it is chosen primarily for its gentle, fresh scent. It is also used because it is excellent for soothing dry skin, for clearing skin infections and for balancing greasy and dry skins. It can help clear other infections, such as thrush and respiratory conditions – and it can be used to support the immune system. Rosewood is a gentle sedative which eases breathing and can help to fight discouragement and nightmares, and it will leave you feeling both emotionally and physically cleansed.

Maximum dose *4 drops in 20ml (0.6fl oz) carrier oil*

Leaves

Plant leaves are where photosynthesis takes place – where the plant produces the energy it needs for life. The essential oils listed below are all extracted from the leaves of their plants and they are linked to the digestive system – stimulating appetites, easing nausea and cooling inflammation.

Lemongrass

Cymbopogon citratus

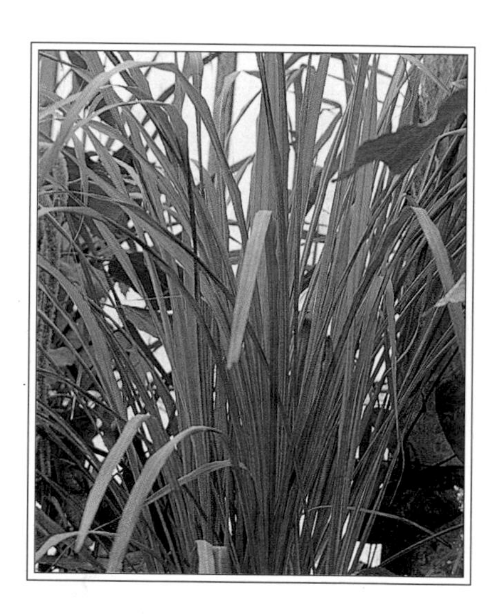

A key ingredient in oriental cooking, Lemongrass is closely associated with the digestive system, helping to ease nausea, gastritis, vomiting, colitis and gastric reflux. When used in a massage blend, the essential oil has the same properties, and is also very useful for easing muscular aches and pains and joint pain associated with some forms of arthritis. More importantly, given its tropical origins, it can keep fleas, lice and mosquitoes at bay. A mild stimulant, Lemongrass is very uplifting, helping people to concentrate and to fight depression. It can occasionally bring on an allergic reaction in some people, so avoid using it if you have very sensitive or damaged skin.

Maximum dose *3 drops in 20ml (0.6fl oz) carrier oil*

Patchouli

Pogostemon cablin

Patchouli has been used in perfumes and incense for generations. It has a cool, leafy and musky scent which helps to stimulate the appetite, relieving nausea and irritable bowel syndrome. It can help to alleviate morning sickness if this continues beyond the first trimester of pregnancy. It helps to cool and relieve acne, eczema, dermatitis and inflamed and cracked skin. It is also used as an aphrodisiac.

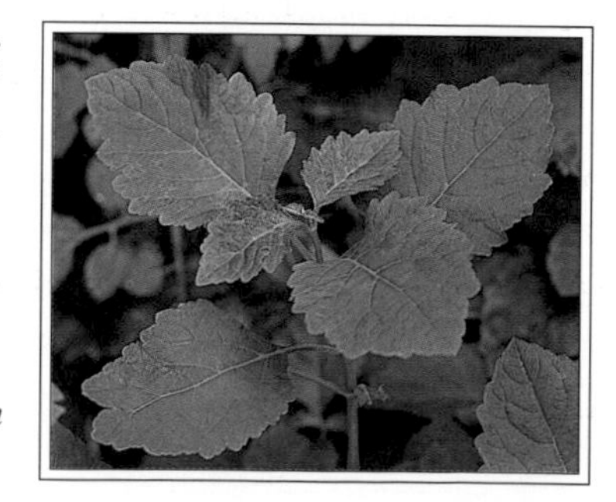

Maximum dose *2 drops in 20ml (0.6fl oz) carrier oil*

Palmarosa

Cymbopogon martini

Palmarosa is an uninspiring-looking grass which is grown in India and Brazil. It has a light, fresh, slightly citrus-like aroma, which seems far too pretty for its qualities. It is effective in the treatment of pelvic inflammatory diseases, cystitis, thrush, colitis, intestinal parasites and ear infections. It also helps other forms of inflammation, like eczema and acne, pharyngitis and even emotional 'inflammation'. Feelings of anger, rage and jealousy all respond to the cooling, refreshing action of Palmarosa.

Maximum dose *3 drops in 20ml (0.6fl oz) carrier oil*

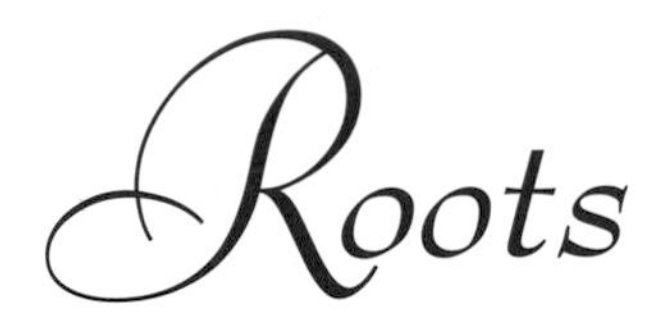

Roots

Earthy and musky, roots tend to have a good grounding effect, inducing a sense of calm and channelling concentration on the here and now. They generally have links to more than one body system, just as roots supply water and strength to the whole plant. These essential oils tend to supply a sense of strength to a blend.

Ginger

Zingiber officinale

Like the root it is distilled from, Ginger essential oil is closely linked with the digestive system, easing nausea, indigestion, diarrhoea and stomach cramps. A warming and invigorating oil, it is excellent for relieving muscular aches and pains and poor circulation. It encourages the quick return to health following strains, sprains and fractures and can ease bronchitis, chesty coughs and colds.

Maximum dose *2 drops in 20ml (0.6fl oz) carrier oil*

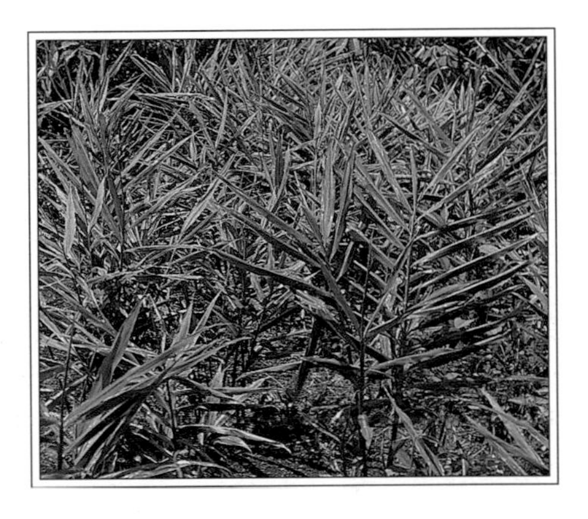

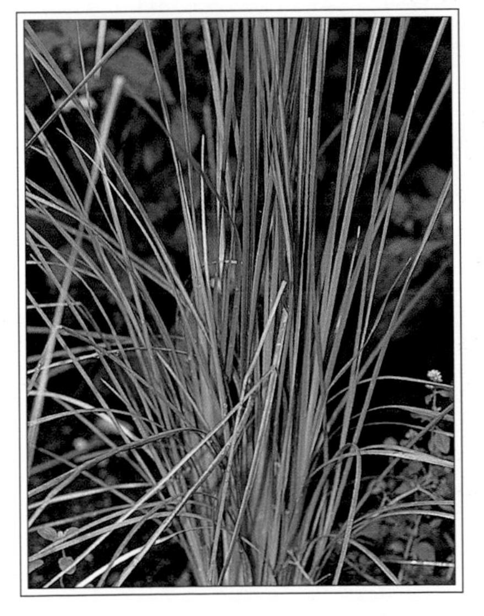

Vetiver

Vetiveria zizanoides

Vetiver has a deep earthy scent and it is a frequent ingredient in men's perfumes. Excellent for relieving muscular aches and pains, it can also be used to clear constipation, colitis and lymphatic congestion. It is reputed to be closely associated with the liver and can sometimes improve liver function in those recovering from alcohol addiction. It is also very closely associated with the reproductive system. It can also prepare the body for conception – regulating the menstrual cycle, increasing fertility in women and increasing potency in men. It is a very supportive oil for those who show no interest in life, feel a lack of security or confidence and are unable to relax.

Maximum dose *2 drops in 20ml (0.6fl oz) carrier oil*

Fruit

Fruit essential oils are widely available and when applied to the skin, they are excellent for lifting spirits, boosting the immune system and refreshing the mind. The little bubbles of liquid stored in citrus fruit peel are the essential oils, and when a recipe calls for the zest of a fruit, it is the essential oil that gives it flavour.

These citrus oils can make your skin marginally more sensitive to sunlight, so do not use more than the recommended number of drops if you are intending to sunbathe, or use a sunbed, within the following twelve hours.

Lemon

Citrus limonum

Lemon is another very effective cleanser which is closely associated with the skin. Acne, bruises, warts, verrucas, cellulite, broken capillaries, scabies, insect bites, rashes, allergic reactions or excessively oily skin will all benefit from the use of Lemon. It is the most effective of all the citrus oils in fighting nausea, halitosis, flatulence, constipation and diarrhoea. It is also good for clearing headaches, and is a good supporting oil for migraine sufferers. Its fresh, zesty scent is a good stimulant, keeping the mind alert and ready for action – dispelling feelings of confusion, anxiety and despair.

Maximum dose *4 drops in 20ml (0.6fl oz) carrier oil*

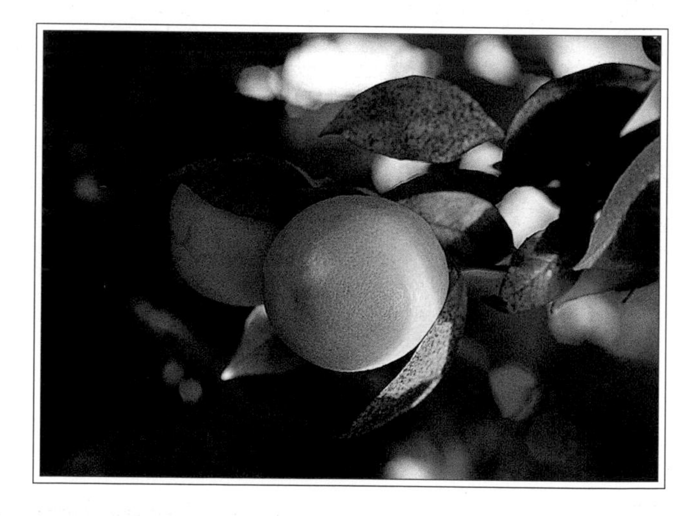

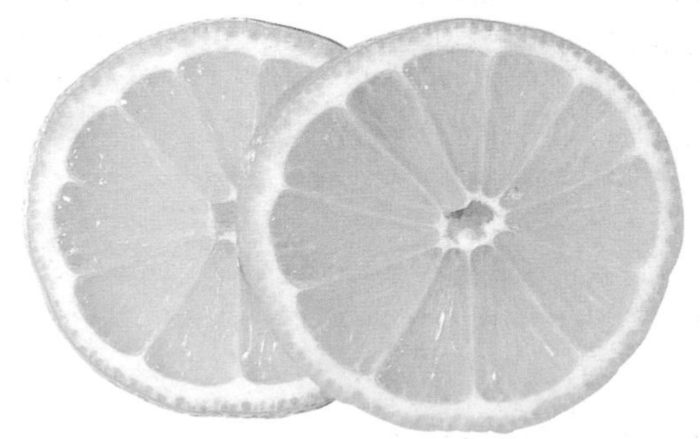

Orange

Citrus aurantium var sinensis

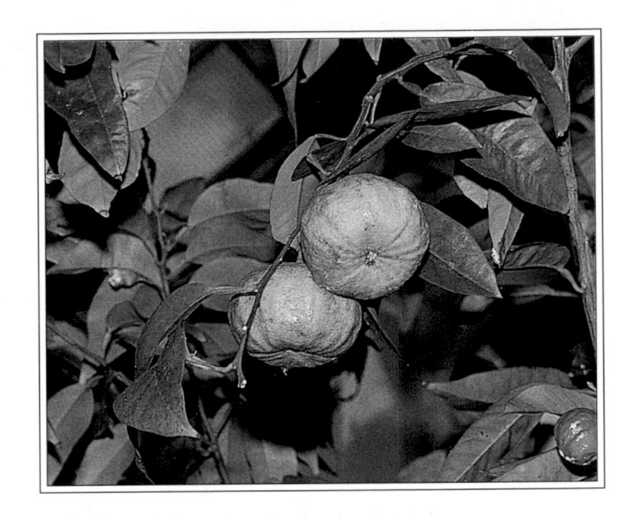

Orange is very useful for those suffering from indigestion, nausea, constipation, gastritis, flatulence or halitosis. It also helps to reduce fluid retention and can be useful in reducing acne, dermatitis and thread veins. Orange is very soothing and uplifting, making it ideal for those who are experiencing feelings of frustration, discouragement and despair. A mild essential oil, it is very effective for use with small children experiencing sleep difficulties, nightmares, indigestion or anxiety.

Maximum dose *4 drops in 20ml (0.6fl oz) carrier oil*

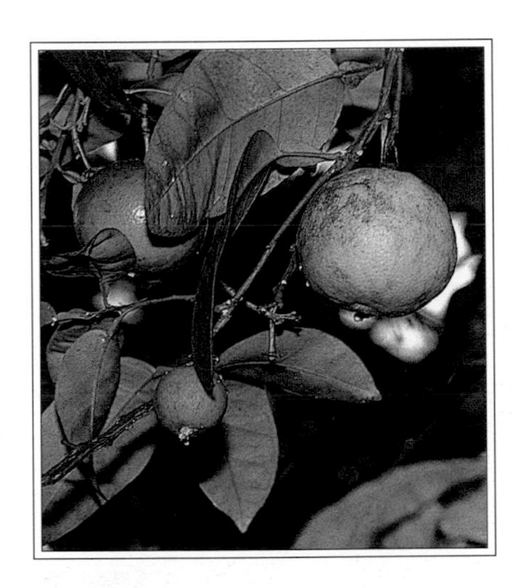

Grapefruit

Citrus paradisi

Grapefruit is an extremely effective cleanser – it helps to reduce fluid retention, making it very useful for cellulite treatments. It will also help indigestion sufferers, and those with flatulence or mild liver and gall bladder problems, and when used in a massage oil, it is a very useful support if you want to beat the winter blues with a detoxification diet. Refreshing and uplifting, it helps to dispel feelings of apathy, resentment, boredom and disinterest.

Maximum dose *4 drops in 20ml (0.6fl oz) carrier oil*

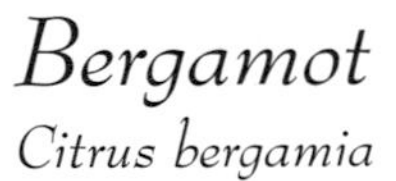

Bergamot

Citrus bergamia

The bitter orange used to flavour Earl Grey tea, Bergamot is closely associated with skin conditions. It can be used to clear acne, boils, eczema, dermatitis and psoriasis, as well as to relieve digestive complaints such as abdominal distension and discomfort, nausea, irritable bowel syndrome, gastroenteritis and flatulence. It is also extremely useful for fighting urogenital, mouth and throat infections. Treat urogenital complaints using Bergamot in bath products, and mouth and throat infections using moisturisers and face oils applied to the face and neck. As a general immune stimulant, Bergamot can relieve feelings of anxiety, depression, restlessness, lethargy and it can reduce stress-related skin conditions.

Maximum dose *4 drops in 20ml (0.6fl oz) carrier oil*

Herbs

Extracted from the leaves and sometimes the flowers of herbaceous perennials, these essential oils can aid the easing of muscular aches and pains. They are also good for clearing the mind, and help to focus you on the task at hand.

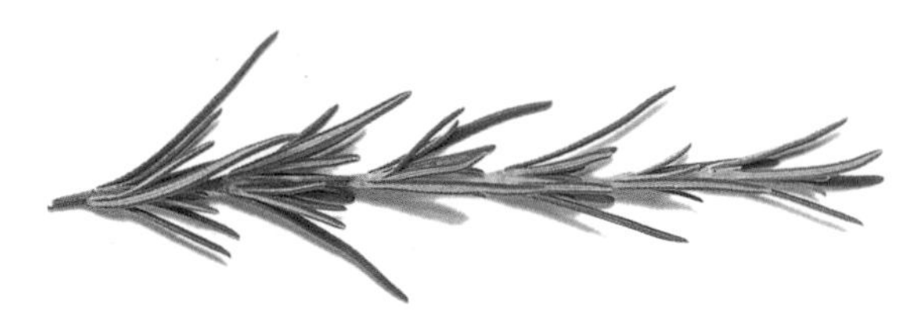

Rosemary

Rosemarinus officinalis

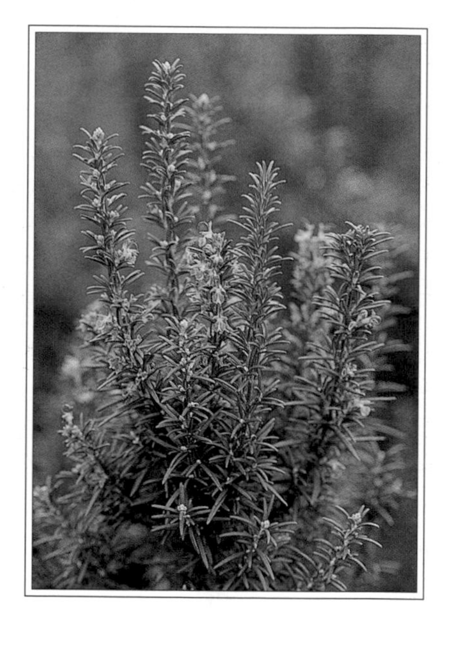

One of the key ingredients of most chest complaint remedies, Rosemary is an extremely strong expectorant; it can help to clear mucus caused by chronic bronchitis, colds and respiratory discomforts. It is closely associated with the easing of muscular aches and pains, sprains, strains and some of the pain associated with arthritic conditions, and it can be used if you are suffering from mental fatigue, have difficulty concentrating, or feel lethargic.

Rosemary helps to raise the blood pressure – so it is useful for low blood pressure sufferers. However, it should be avoided if you have high blood pressure, epilepsy and fevers, or if you are pregnant or breast-feeding.

Maximum dose *2 drops in 20ml (0.6fl oz) carrier oil*

Yarrow

Achillea millefolium

The bright blue colour of the Yarrow essential oil marks it as having the same key ingredient as German Chamomile. It has excellent anti-inflammatory properties. I have seen it work extremely effectively in easing dermatitis, eczema, allergic skin reactions and other inflammatory conditions. These include muscular aches and pains, rheumatoid arthritis, cystitis, gastritis and colitis. A gentle sedative and pain killer, it is extremely useful for those suffering from chronic fatigue, anxiety, insomnia, frustration and anger.

Maximum dose *2 drops in 20ml (0.6fl oz) carrier oil*

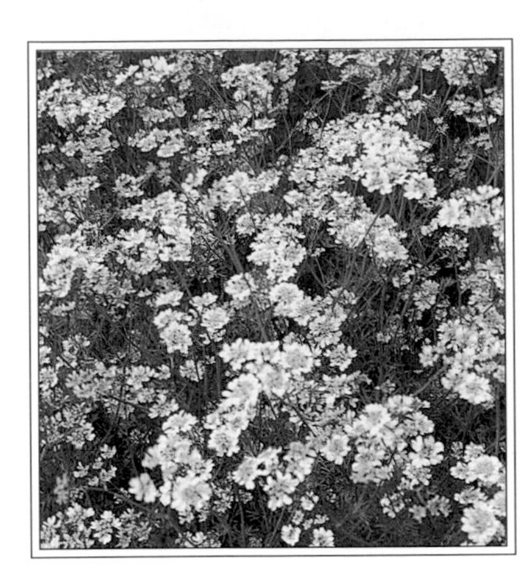

Coriander

Coriandrum sativum

This warm, spicy essential oil is closely linked to the stomach and intestines. It can help relieve nervous indigestion, nausea, vomiting and constipation – either as an inhalant or as part of a moisturiser, massage blend or perfume. It also has a reputation as an aphrodisiac.

Maximum dose *3 drops in 20ml (0.6fl oz) carrier oil*

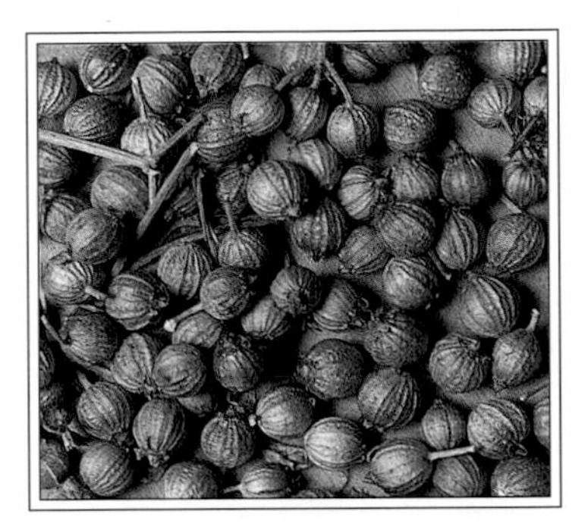

Peppermint

Mentha piperita

Strongly associated with the digestive system, when used in a massage oil Peppermint is excellent for soothing the spasms of colic, diarrhoea, gastritis, irritable bowel syndrome, stomach cramps, vomiting and indigestion. It also helps clear flatulence and halitosis, nausea and toothache. Peppermint smells and feels cool when applied, but its overall effect is the opposite, which makes it useful for easing muscular aches and pains, poor circulation and the discomforts of colds, headaches, neuralgia and even hangovers! A refreshing oil, it helps to improve memory and ease mental fatigue.

Maximum dose *2 drops in 20ml (0.6fl oz) carrier oil*

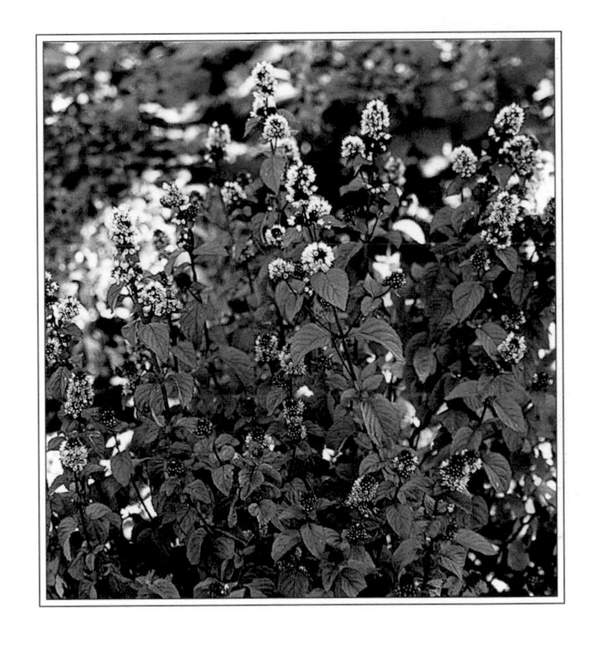

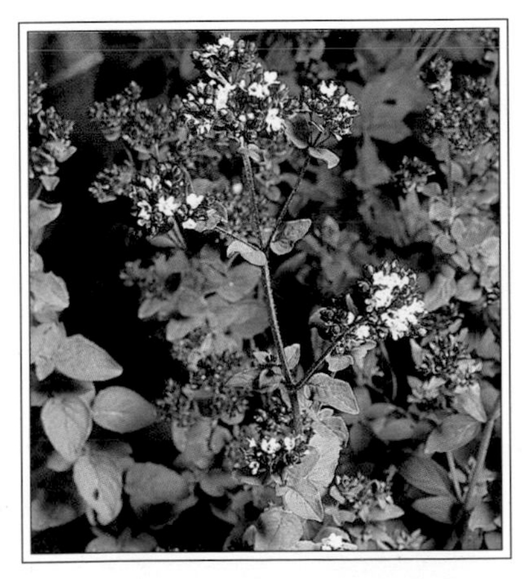

Marjoram

Origanum marjorana

This gentle herb is an extremely effective remedy for muscular aches and pains and muscle spasms. As part of an abdominal massage, or in bubble baths and shower gels, it can aid constipation, soothe joints troubled by arthritis and relieve colic and colitis. Marjoram is also good for relieving high blood pressure and migraines, and it is an effective sedative. Try it when anxiety, panic or grief are disturbing your sleep.

Maximum dose *3 drops in 20ml (0.6fl oz) carrier oil*

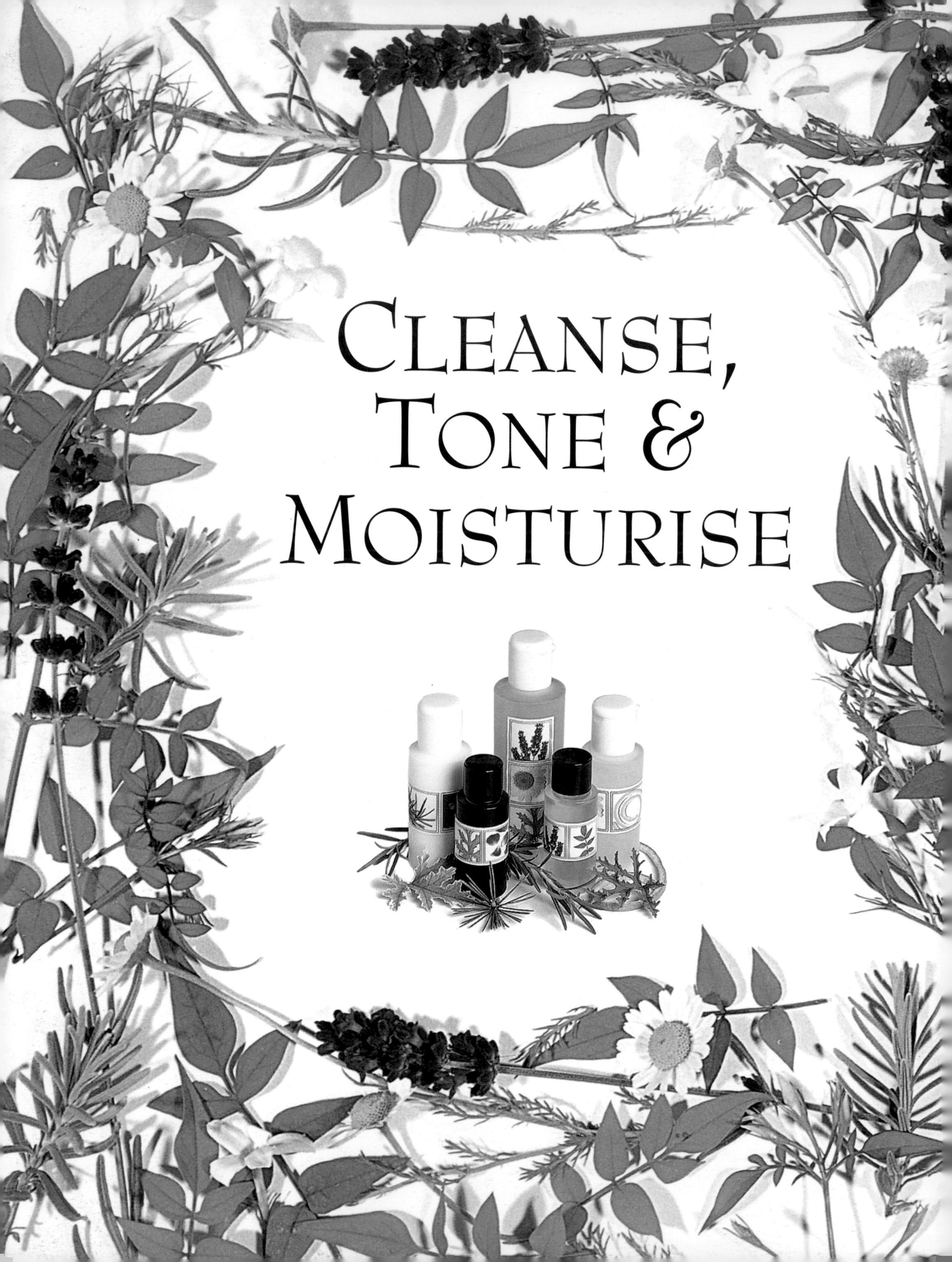

Cleanse, Tone & Moisturise

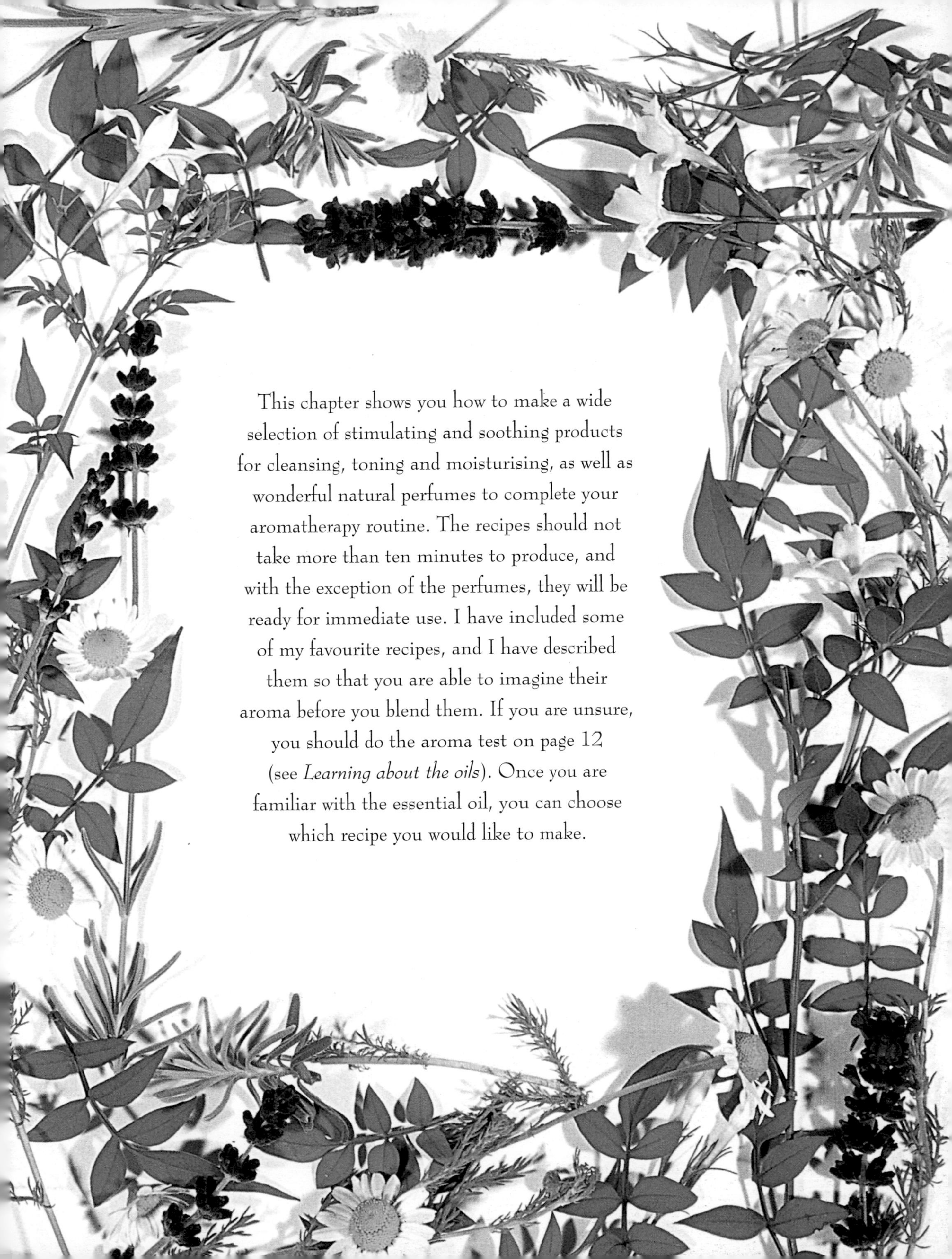

This chapter shows you how to make a wide selection of stimulating and soothing products for cleansing, toning and moisturising, as well as wonderful natural perfumes to complete your aromatherapy routine. The recipes should not take more than ten minutes to produce, and with the exception of the perfumes, they will be ready for immediate use. I have included some of my favourite recipes, and I have described them so that you are able to imagine their aroma before you blend them. If you are unsure, you should do the aroma test on page 12 (see *Learning about the oils*). Once you are familiar with the essential oil, you can choose which recipe you would like to make.

Materials

Glass jars and bottles Various shapes and sizes are needed for your blends. Glass is better than plastic, as it can be sterilised at a high temperature after use, and you can therefore recycle any beautiful bottles you find. Amber glass jars and bottles are usually available from your local chemist.

Plastic bottles Plastic bottles of various shapes and sizes are best for blends that will be placed near the bath or shower. Containers with flip-top caps, pump actions or sprays are suitable. Be careful about recycling them however, as plastic can retain traces of essential oils. Do not use plastic bottles which have contained medication.

Glass mixing bowl and glass rod A glass mixing bowl or jug and a glass rod are best for blending, as they can be cleaned properly after use. If you don't have a glass rod, a metal spoon can be used instead.

Unperfumed, lanolin-free bubble baths, shower gels, shampoos, conditioners, moisturisers and cleansers Various such products are now available. They often have labels indicating they can be used on infants, or on sensitive or damaged skin. You should avoid perfume-based products. Lanolin, a waxy product found on sheep's wool, also causes some sensitivity in those who are allergic to wool, or have very sensitive skin, so is best avoided.

Grapeseed oil This good, all-purpose carrier oil is ideal as a base for massage blends or bath oils. It has a light, non-greasy texture, so it will not feel sticky.

Avocado oil This carrier oil is heavier than Jojoba and is therefore appropriate for a drier, more mature skin. It is useful for anti-ageing blends.

Sweet Almond oil A good all-round carrier oil which is also useful for massage blends.

Calendula oil This light oil is not as greasy as Sweet Almond oil. It is wonderful for treating scar tissue and reducing the size and appearance of stretch marks, and can help to heal skin marked by severe acne. If you find that it doesn't moisturise your skin as much as you would like, blend it with equal portions of Jojoba or Grapeseed oil.

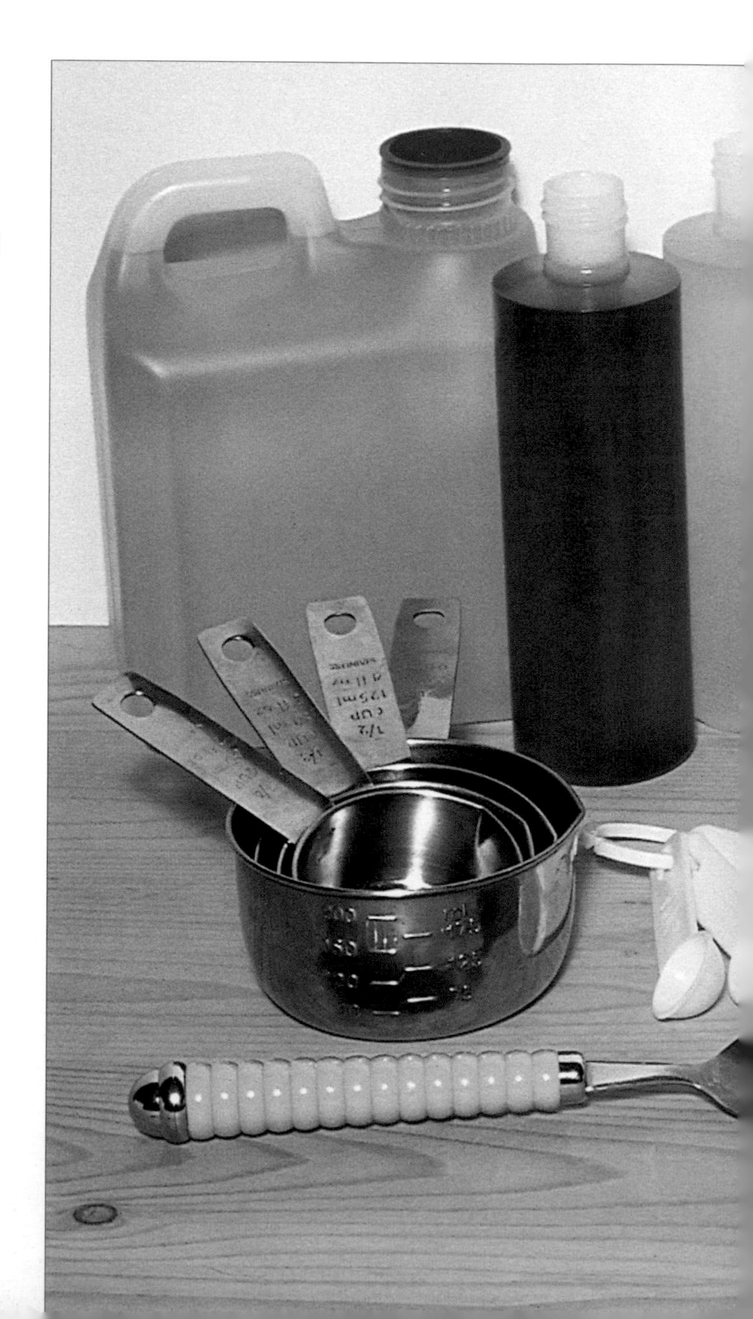

Jojoba oil Jojoba is technically a wax, bought in liquid form. It is an enriching carrier oil and a wonderful base for face products – either as a face oil itself, or used sparingly to enhance a moisturiser.

Flower waters These are a by-product of the distillation of essential oils and they smell slightly of their floral origins. Gently astringent, they can be used on their own as effective toners. Rose Water smells pleasant and is available from most pharmacies. Orange Flower water (Neroli) also has a pleasant smell. Both are useful bases for perfumes. Lavender water is an acquired taste and might be best left alone.

Surgical spirit/alcohol Surgical spirit or alcohol can be used to fix perfumes. If you are using alcohol, vodka is the most appropriate as it has no scent of its own.

Measuring cups, jugs or spoons These are used to measure liquid base products. A glass measuring jug would be appropriate, although a plastic one is fine, as long as the essential oils are not placed in it.

Metal spoon For blending when you don't have access to a glass rod. This is easier to clean than plastic or wood.

Essential oils See recipes.

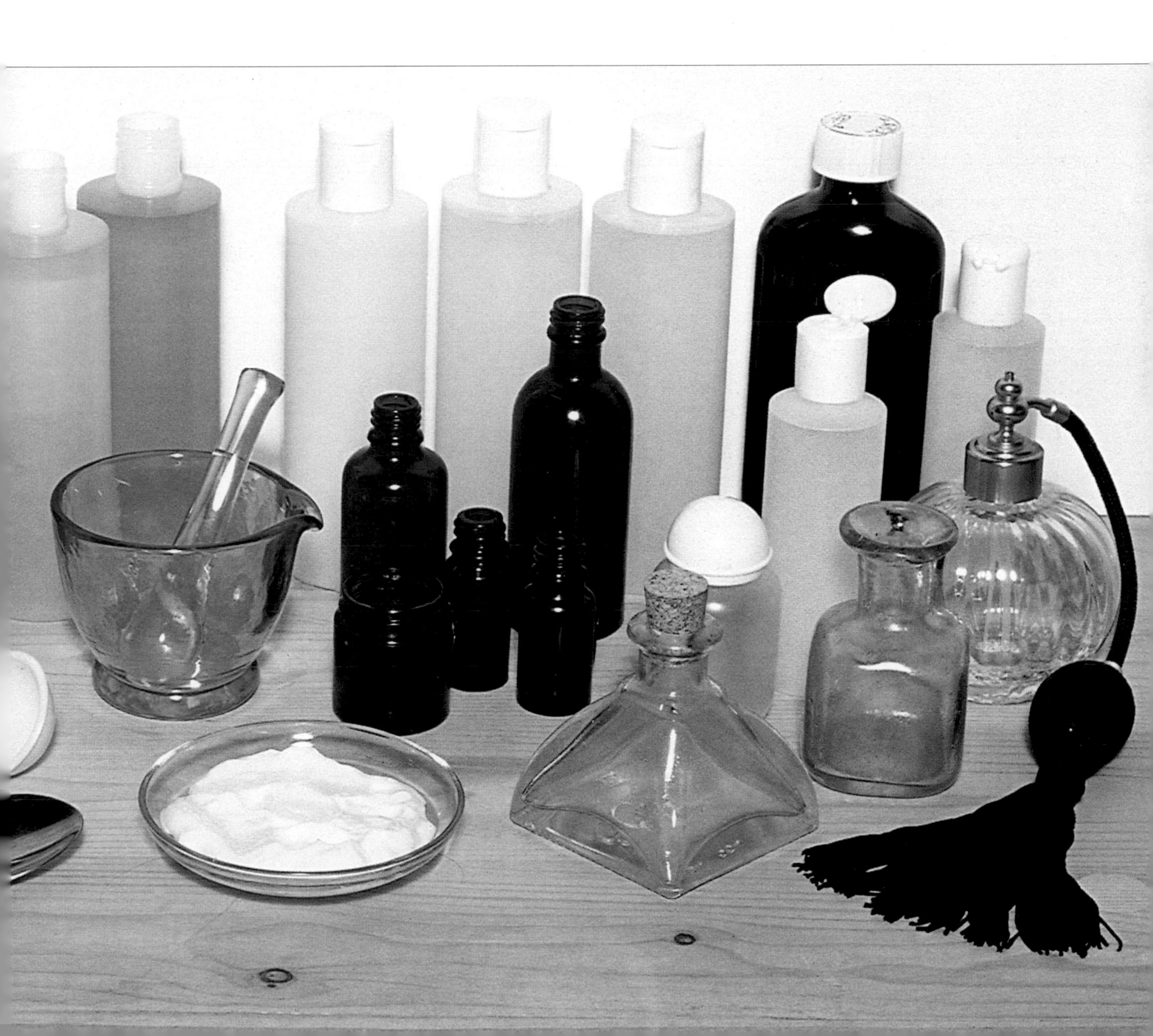

Techniques

Shampoos, face oils, cleansers and toners, shower gels, bubble baths, moisturisers and massage oils can be made quickly and easily. Use an unperfumed base that relates to the item you want to make. I am making a shampoo here, and have chosen an unperfumed, lanolin-free shampoo base.

The amount of essential oils added depends on the quantity of base product used. As a guide, for a total of 20ml (0.6fl oz) of liquid base product, use 8 drops of essential oils. Use 20 drops for every 50g (1.8oz) of cream base.

You can use just one essential oil, or choose several. Here, I use a total of 100ml (3.2fl oz) of shampoo base and 40 drops from a selection of three essential oils.

Perfumes are made in the same way, substituting flower water and surgical spirit or alcohol in place of the base product. To make perfumes, use surgical spirit or alcohol at Step 1 and the flower water at Step 4. You will notice that you use fewer drops of essential oil for perfumes; this is because the essential oils don't mix as well with water and alcohol as they do with carrier oils. At these lower levels, you are unlikely to get an adverse skin reaction.

Storing finished products

Your finished products have a shelf life of around one month to six weeks. This can be extended by an extra two weeks if the products are stored in a cool location, such as a fridge. Although the perfume should remain beyond this period, the blends are unlikely to be fully effective in therapeutic terms.

You will need

Base liquid or cream or
Surgical spirit /Alcohol and Flower water
Glass bowl ~ Measuring jug
Essential oil(s) ~ Glass rod
Sterilised bottle

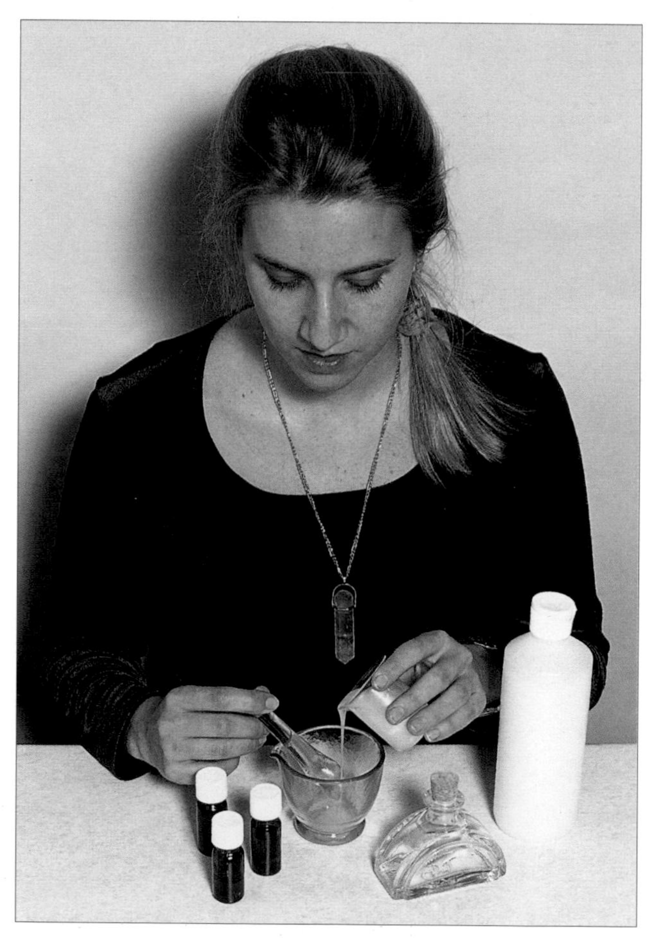

1. Check the recipe and measure out the base product. Pour half of the quantity into a glass bowl. For perfume, pour all the alcohol into the bowl.

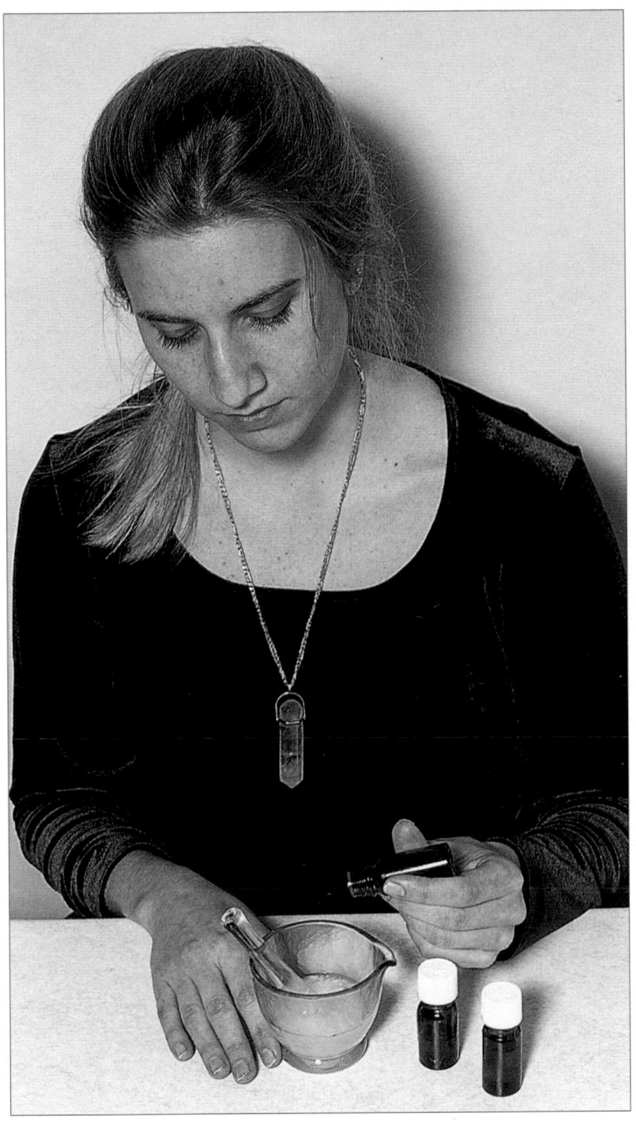

2. Carefully add 8 drops of essential oil(s) for every 20ml (0.6fl oz) of base liquid, or 20 drops for every 50g (1.8oz) of base cream.

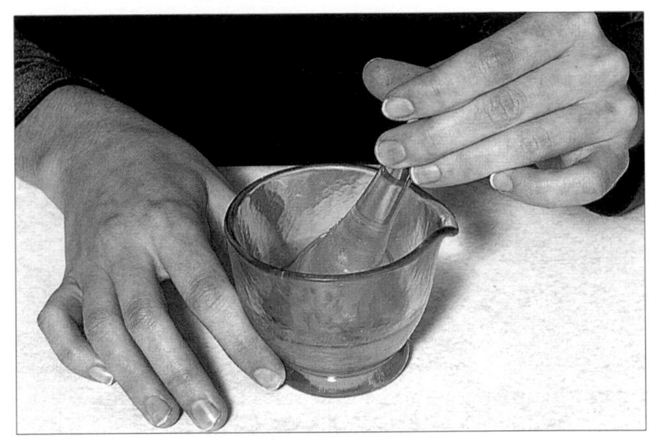

3. Mix well using a glass rod or metal spoon, for 30 seconds or until all the oils are thoroughly mixed in to the base product.

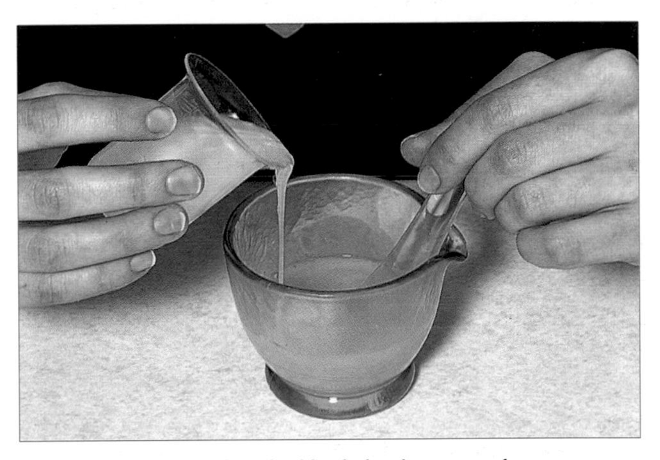

4. Pour in the other half of the base product. Mix well, until the oils are thoroughly mixed in. For perfumes, add the flower water at this stage.

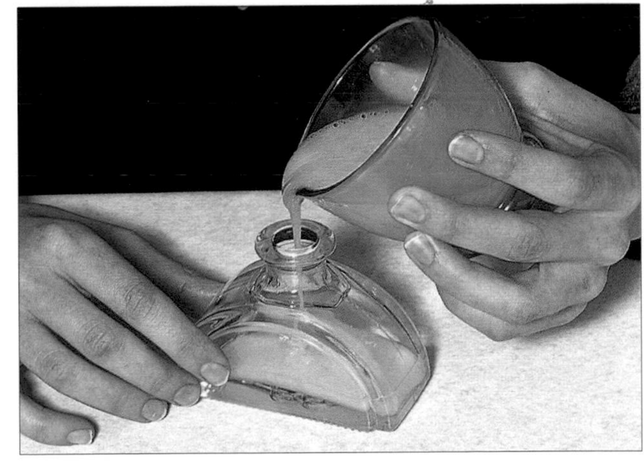

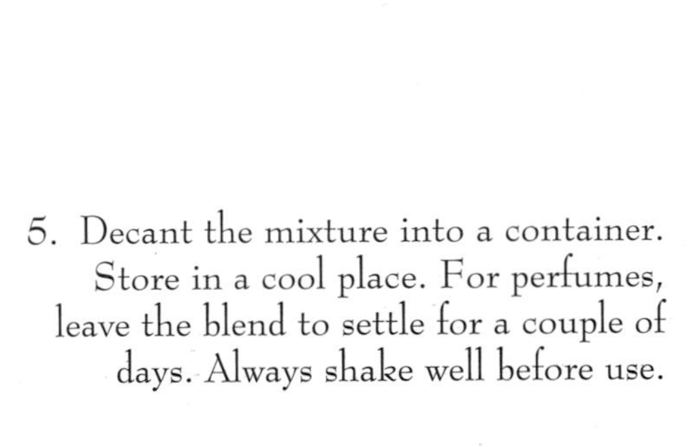

5. Decant the mixture into a container. Store in a cool place. For perfumes, leave the blend to settle for a couple of days. Always shake well before use.

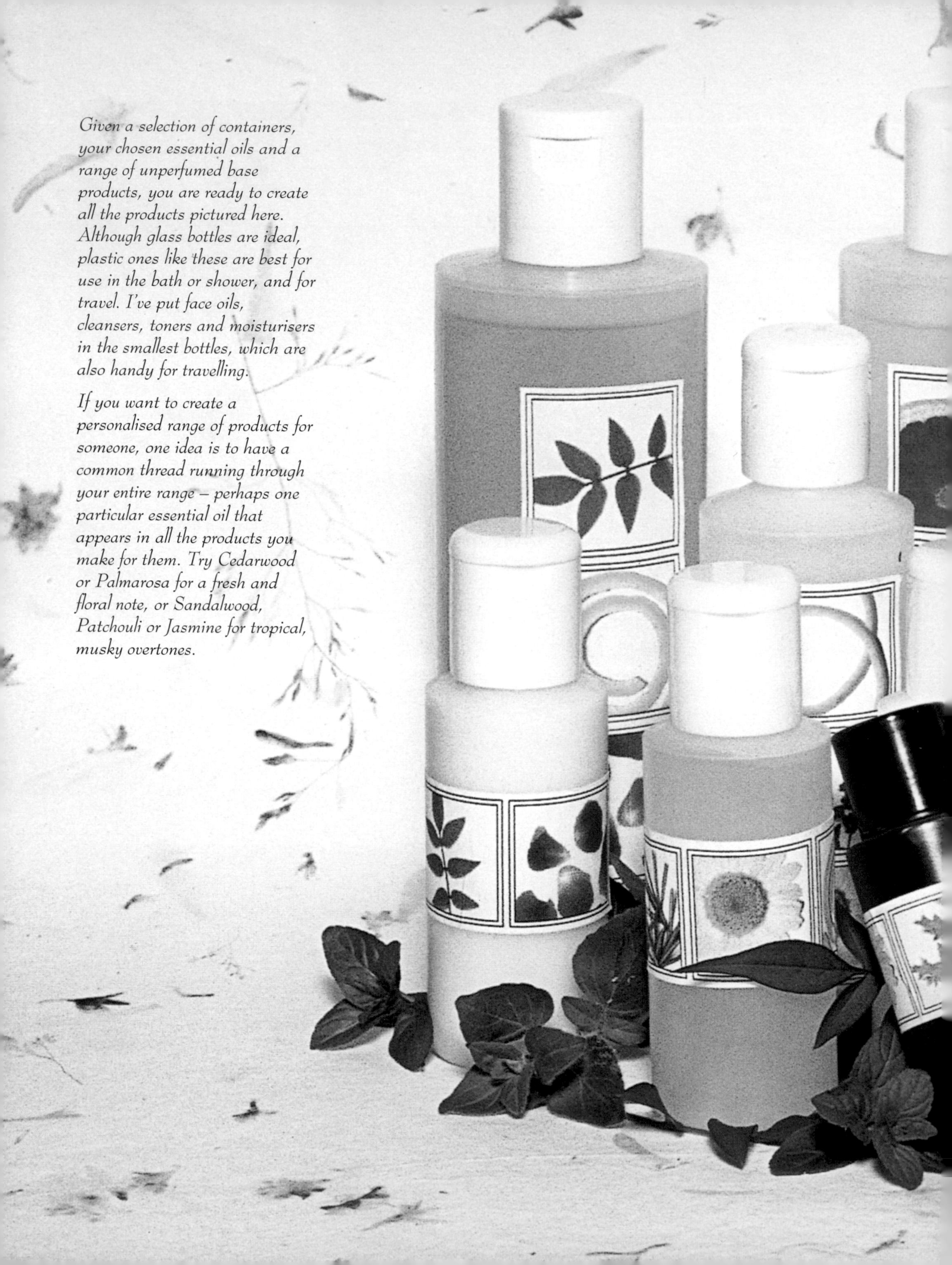

Given a selection of containers, your chosen essential oils and a range of unperfumed base products, you are ready to create all the products pictured here. Although glass bottles are ideal, plastic ones like these are best for use in the bath or shower, and for travel. I've put face oils, cleansers, toners and moisturisers in the smallest bottles, which are also handy for travelling.

If you want to create a personalised range of products for someone, one idea is to have a common thread running through your entire range – perhaps one particular essential oil that appears in all the products you make for them. Try Cedarwood or Palmarosa for a fresh and floral note, or Sandalwood, Patchouli or Jasmine for tropical, musky overtones.

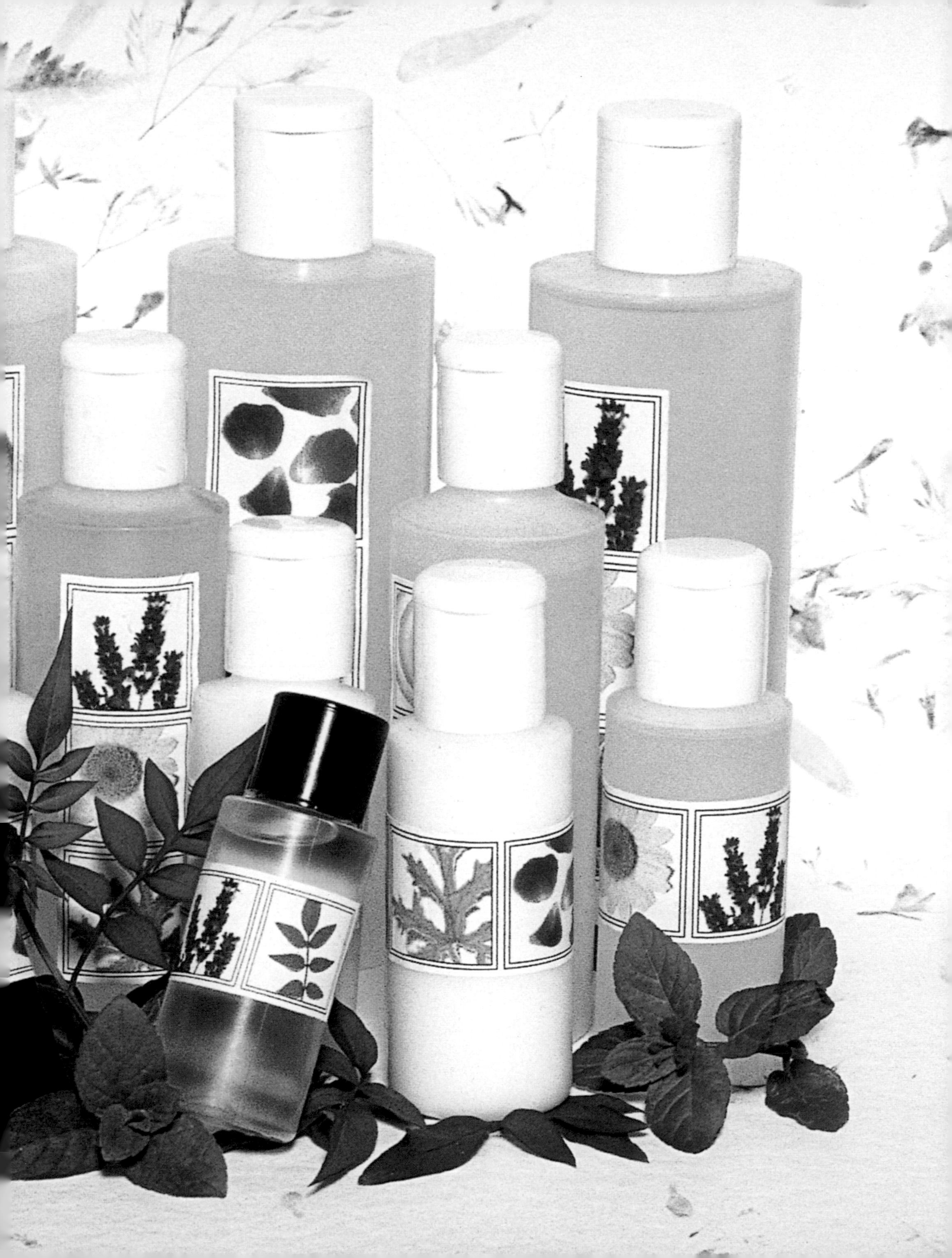

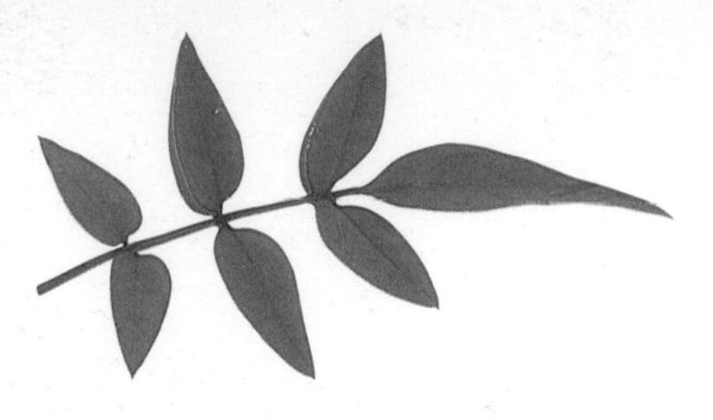

Recipes

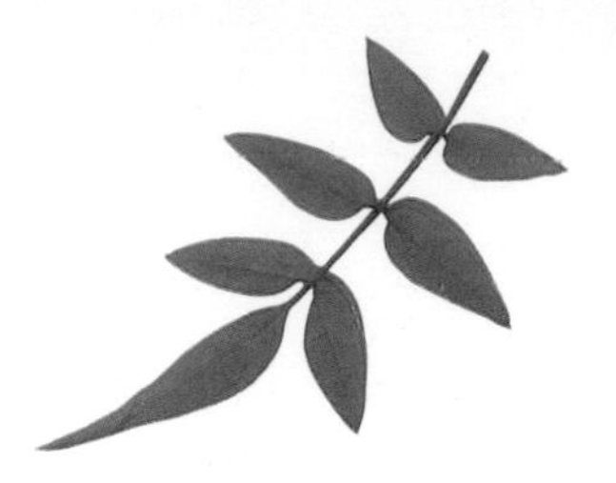

Cleansers and Toners

Cleansers and toners can enhance the effects of aromatherapy face oils and moisturisers, and speed up the healing rate, when used in your daily routine. Use an unperfumed cleanser as a base.

Cleansers remove trapped dirt, cleanse the skin and calm and soothe any inflamed areas. They are particularly effective when used with essential oils which have strong antiseptic qualities, such as Lavender, Bergamot, Geranium and Grapefruit. Anti-inflammatories such as Yarrow and Chamomile are excellent, as are oils such as Cedarwood, Sandalwood, Frankincense, Patchouli, Benzoin, Rosewood and Rose, which all help to heal skin conditions.

The above oils are excellent too when used in toner recipes, although the more astringent ones are better for particularly oily skin – Lemon, Peppermint, Rosemary and Lemongrass. These can be blended in unscented toners or, for the best results, use flower waters such as Orange Blossom or Rose Water. Rose Water blended with Witch Hazel is a good base for an oily skin. The Witch Hazel gives the Rose Water a more astringent and antiseptic quality. Plain Rose Water is more appropriate for anyone with dry or sensitive skin.

Eau de Cologne Toner

The recipe for Eau de Cologne is centuries old. This version uses four of the original ingredients to make a refreshing, stimulating and astringent toner. If you have very dry or sensitive skin, you might want to reduce the amount of Rosemary to 2 drops and add an extra drop each of Neroli and Lavender.

Neroli 1 drop
Lavender 2 drops
Rosemary 4 drops
Bergamot 3 drops
40ml (1.3fl oz) Rose Water or unscented toner

Citrus Cleanser

A woody, citrus-like, mildly astringent blend which is excellent for combination skin – it will help to balance out patches of dry and oily skin.

Grapefruit 4 drops
Geranium 2 drops
Cedarwood 3 drops
50g (1.8oz) cleanser

Forest Toner

A soothing blend which cools and calms the skin. It can also help to reduce the inflammation and infection associated with acne.

Bergamot 7 drops
Sandalwood 5 drops
Lavender 3 drops
40ml (1.3fl oz) Rose Water or unscented toner

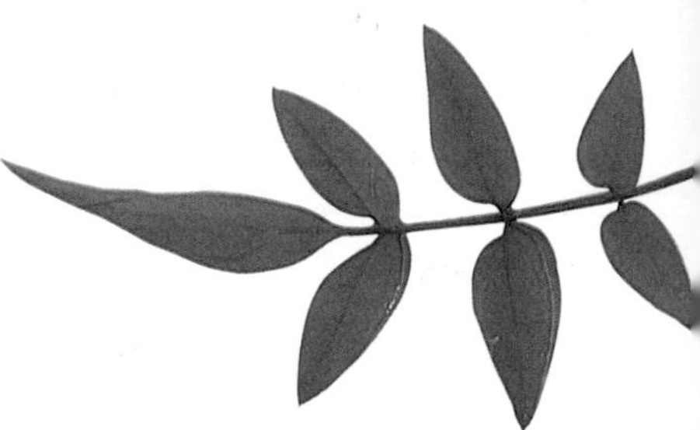

Cheer Up Cleanser

This is a delicate blend which raises the spirits and improves circulation. Rosewood and Grapefruit are both mild astringents and together with Palmarosa they will improve the colour and texture of the skin.

Palmarosa 3 drops
Rosewood 4 drops
Grapefruit 3 drops
50g (1.8oz) cleanser

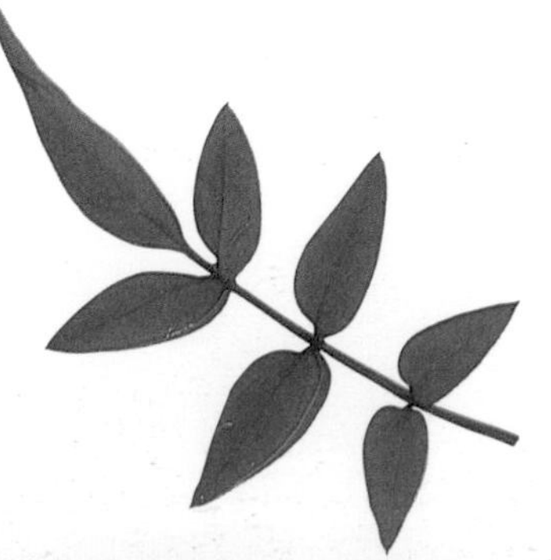

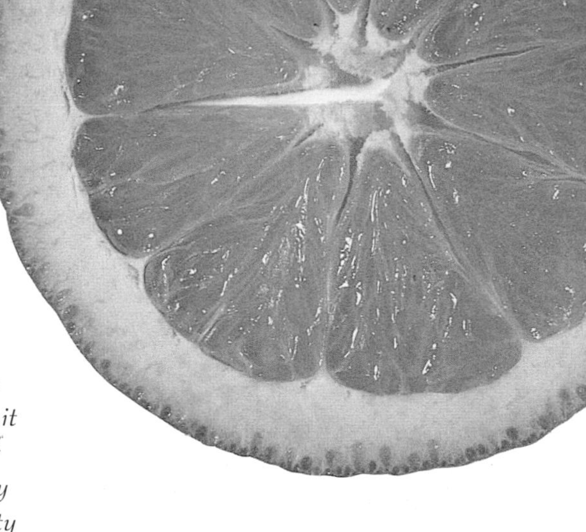

Moisturisers

Moisturisers are one of the easiest cosmetics to enhance with essential oils. There is a large range of lanolin-free, fragrance-free, hypoallergenic products available. A moisturiser's job is to soothe dry skin, reduce fine lines and provide a little additional help at weatherproofing. You can enhance the effects of your moisturiser, not only with essential oils, but also by adding a little Jojoba oil – 5ml (0.2fl oz) for every 50g (1.8oz) of moisturiser – or an Evening Primrose oil capsule to the blend.

Don't forget, you can adapt these recipes to use them with a liquid base – a bubble bath, shampoo or shower gel. Simply increase the liquid base to 60ml (1.8fl oz) and use the same recipe given here.

After Gardening

This aromatic herbaceous moisturiser brings the garden into the home, reminding us of how plants can be beneficial in a variety of ways. Lavender has antiseptic properties and will soothe cuts, grazes, insect bites or stings. Lemon is a mild astringent and Marjoram is wonderful for aching muscles and joints.

Lavender 3 drops
Lemon 2 drops
Marjoram 3 drops
50g (1.8oz) moisturiser

The Orange Tree

A light blend which smells like a citrus grove – the blossom and fruit of the orange tree, plus a hint of wood. An excellent remedy for dry skin, for those experiencing anxiety or for anyone unable to fully express their emotions.

Orange 6 drops
Neroli 4 drops
Sandalwood 10 drops
50g (1.8oz) moisturiser

After-Sun

This soothes burnt skin and is extremely useful when used as an after-sun cream. It can also reduce uncomfortable, dry, scaly eczema patches. As an added bonus, it seems to keep mosquitoes at bay too!

Yarrow 4 drops
Lavender 8 drops
Cedarwood 4 drops
Bergamot 3 drops
50 g (1.8oz) moisturiser

Tropical Holiday

A warm and soothing blend which smells like sunlight in the rainforest after a storm has blown over. It is wonderful for dry or blemished skin.

Patchouli 6 drops
Palmarosa 7 drops
Lemon 7 drops
50g (1.8oz) moisturiser

Sleepy Time

As well as being a great moisturiser for cracked skin, this is an effective remedy for those experiencing constipation, insomnia or nightmares. A favourite blend with children, the vanilla-like smell of Benzoin, and the fruity orange aroma, make this a familiar and comfortable fragrance. These oils can also be used in a bubble bath.

Orange 9 drops
Benzoin 6 drops
Roman Chamomile 5 drops
50g (1.8oz) moisturiser

Aching Joints

This is an excellent moisturiser for anyone who has aching joints. It offers a little pain relief, and it will warm the hands and soothe the skin. Add a capsule of Evening Primrose oil to the blend and you will have a lovely rich moisturiser which should improve the condition of your hands.

Roman Chamomile 4 drops
Yarrow 4 drops
Lavender 6 drops
Rose 2 drops
50g (1.8oz) moisturiser

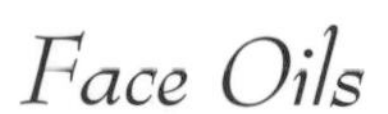

Face Oils

A certain amount of oil is needed in our skin to keep it waterproof, weatherproof and generally in good condition. A face oil can help. Sparingly applied, the right blend can balance adolescent skin – clearing it and leaving it supple and reasonably unblemished.

Jojoba oil helps to maintain more mature skin, and can reduce fine lines. Jojoba oil is also particularly effective for blemished or combination skin. Its chemical structure is similar to that of sebum, the skin's naturally occurring oil. Sebum dissolves in Jojoba, so by applying it you can help to loosen any dirt trapped in the pores.

Avocado oil is absorbed into drier, finer skin quickly. Its richer, heavier structure means that it is also extremely good as a moisturiser and it is an excellent base under make-up. However, I recommend that you wait at least fifteen minutes after moisturising before applying any make-up.

Where the skin is scarred – from chicken pox, acne, cuts or more severe wounds – try using Calendula oil as a carrier. In many cases, it can significantly reduce the appearance of scar tissue, softening and encouraging the skin's normal growth.

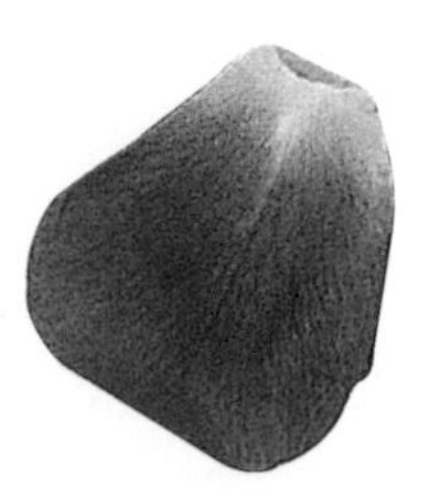

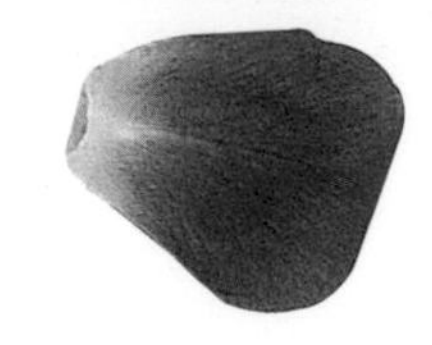

Clarity

This blend is wonderful for adolescent skin which is affected by hormonal changes, and it is popular with teenage males. It smells clean and musky, like a gentle cologne, and makes a nice change from the antiseptic smell of medicinal products.

Lavender 5 drops
Lemon 3 drops
Sandalwood 2 drops
25ml (0.8fl oz) Jojoba oil

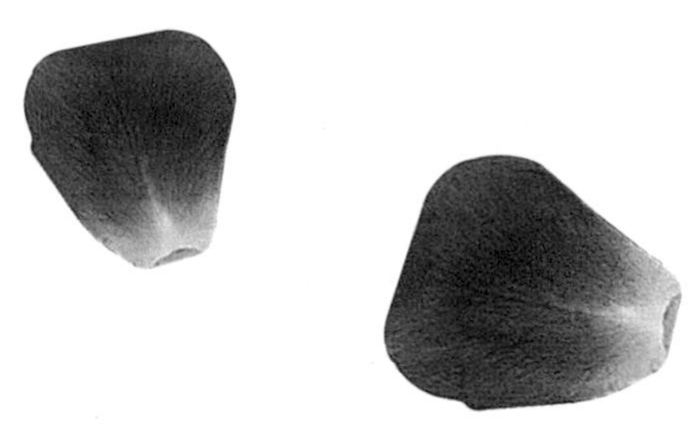

Mirth

'I have, but wherefore I know not/ Lost all my mirth.' Poor Hamlet, he didn't have access to this recipe. When you are having trouble summoning up the energy to be cheerful, it's time to bring a little sweetness into your life. This will leave you feeling on top of the world, whilst also helping to clear minor skin complaints and ease chest infections. It can also help to reduce high blood pressure.

Benzoin 2 drops
Rose 1 drop
Rosewood 2 drops
Palmarosa 3 drops
20ml (0.6fl oz) Jojoba oil

Eraser

I sometimes think of this as nature's bottle of correction fluid – it really does help to soothe and soften scar tissue. It also heals cracked and dry skin, leaving it supple and unblemished.

Benzoin 3 drops
Frankincense 2 drops
Sandalwood 2 drops
Rose 1 drop
20ml (0.6fl oz) Calendula oil

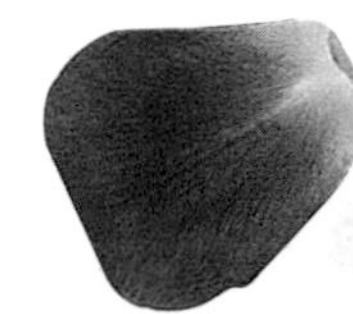

Preservation

A wonderful blend for itching skin and dry eczema or dermatitis, this also doubles as a great after-sun blend if used in a moisturiser. It helps to heal the skin, keeps it moist and stops it itching.

German Chamomile 2 drops
Lavender 4 drops
Cedarwood 3 drops
25ml (0.8fl oz) Grapeseed oil or unperfumed moisturiser

Rejuvenation

This delicate blend is excellent for dry and wrinkled skin, leaving it moist and younger looking. It also smells heavenly – like a flower garden at night, inducing relaxation and sleep if used at bedtime.

Frankincense 4 drops
Rose 2 drops
Neroli 2 drops
20ml (0.6fl oz) Avocado oil

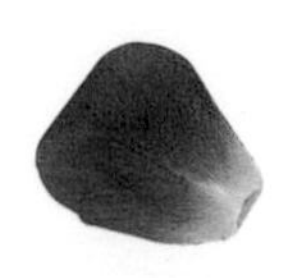

Shampoos

Essential oils can be extremely beneficial when used on the scalp and hair. Different blends can improve blood circulation, make hair shinier, ease dandruff or help combat head lice – and the fragrance will linger in your hair and in the bathroom.

To give your hair the equivalent of a spa holiday, make up the same blend in a carrier oil such as Grapeseed, to make a deep-conditioning treatment. Apply this to your dry hair, wrap it in plastic or in a plastic shower cap, then wrap a towel around your head and leave it for an hour. After an hour, add enough shampoo to the hair to raise a mild lather, then add water and shampoo as normal. This will add extra shine to your hair.

Don't forget, you can also blend essential oils in conditioners, to complete the healthy hair picture. Either stick to the same oils and recipes as for shampoos, or adapt them a bit. Try Flower Garden without the Rosemary, mixed in an unperfumed conditioner.

Flower Garden

An uplifting and energising blend that will bring gloss to your hair, a tingle to your scalp and a smile to your lips.

Geranium 2 drops
Jasmine 2 drops
Lemon 2 drops
Rosemary 2 drops
20ml (0.6fl oz) shampoo

Zest

An energising blend which improves blood circulation to the scalp, leaving you awake and refreshed. Improving circulation has been known to slow down hair loss.

Grapefruit 3 drops
Peppermint 3 drops
Lavender 2 drops
20ml (0.6fl oz) shampoo

Moss

A cool, green, citrus-like blend which will help to clear your head. It will leave you feeling calm and centred throughout the day.

Bergamot 3 drops
Lemongrass 2 drops
Lavender 2 drops
Palmarosa 2 drops
25ml (0.8fl oz) shampoo

Spicy

A spicy, musky shampoo which will leave both you and your bathroom smelling very sultry indeed! With just a hint of innocent Orange, it is a soothing blend.

Coriander 3 drops
Sandalwood 3 drops
Orange 2 drops
20ml (0.6fl oz) shampoo

Circulation

This is quite a strong blend which can help improve blood circulation to the scalp. It can also be used to combat dandruff and dry, flaky skin. Those prone to dandruff may find that using a capful of vinegar in the after-shampoo rinse water will improve the condition of their scalp.

Bergamot 5 drops
Rosemary 2 drops
Lavender 3 drops
25ml (0.8fl oz) shampoo

Strength

This shampoo is a treat for anyone with fine, fragile hair, as the oils have cytophylactic properties (they encourage healthy cell growth). For the best results, before shampooing make up the same blend in a carrier oil such as Grapeseed. Apply a deep-conditioning treatment as described above, then shampoo using this recipe. This will condition your hair and add extra shine.

Sandalwood 2 drops
Frankincense 2 drops
Bergamot 2 drops
Lavender 2 drops
20ml (0.6fl oz) shampoo

Bubble Baths

When things get on top of you, there is nothing quite like a good soak in a hot tub with a good book or some soft music – up to your neck in bubbles. It is relaxing, soothing and uplifting, especially if the bath is perfumed with scented oils, specially chosen for their restorative properties. The following recipes will add a little something to your pleasure, and leave you feeling calm, refreshed and ready to conquer the world.

The recipes here focus on some of the more exotic essential oils, mainly because I am bored with all the commercial bubble baths containing Lavender, Geranium and Ylang Ylang.

If you want a more zesty, energising blend, try creating your own recipe. Start with three essential oils that make you feel refreshed and lively (for a 'morning' type of scent, make one of them a citrus oil – but check that you are not sensitive to these first.) Check the maximum doses for the oils on pages 14–25, then blend accordingly. Try adding your essential oils one drop at a time (one drop of oil A, followed by one of B, and so on), mixing well and then smelling the blend before you add more. This will take longer, but it gives you a clear idea of how just one drop can make a huge difference to how you feel about your creation.

Water Sprite

A tropical blend which should get you going on those cold, grey winter mornings. Lemongrass is great for muscular aches and pains, Coriander will give your immune system a boost and Jasmine regulates hormonal imbalances. This bubble bath smells gorgeous and it can also be used as a perfume. Reduce the dosage of Lemongrass and Jasmine if you have a sensitive skin, as they can sometimes cause an uncomfortable reaction.

Lemongrass 3 drops
Jasmine 2 drops
Coriander 3 drops
20ml (0.6fl oz) bubble bath

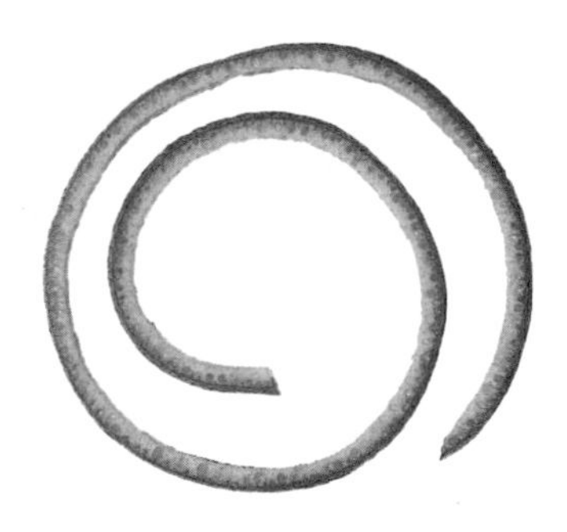

Miracle Worker

When you need to create miracles tomorrow, but can't quite face up to them today, try this blend. Frankincense helps you to breathe calmly and deeply, Ginger settles the butterflies in your stomach and Neroli lifts your spirits and combats shock. The result – a clear head and calm mind.

Frankincense 4 drops
Ginger 2 drops
Neroli 2 drops
20ml (0.6fl oz) bubble bath

Tranquillity

Try this one in the evening – the ingredients will help you sleep. Marjoram and Yarrow are both excellent for muscular aches and pains, especially after heavy exercise. Geranium is uplifting and can promise pleasant dreams. All are good for the skin, especially if it is dry.

Marjoram 3 drops
Yarrow 3 drops
Geranium 2 drops
20ml (0.6fl oz) bubble bath

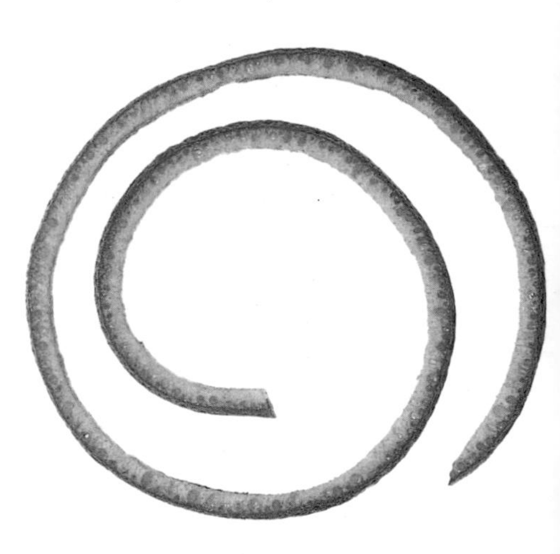

Zen

Not quite a minimalist blend, but the effects leave you completely calm, with a clutter-free mind and a beatific smile on your face. It's good for muscular aches and pains, sinusitis, minor chest complaints and for when your immune system needs a bit of a boost. Also excellent for keeping mosquitoes at bay.

Coriander 3 drops
Patchouli 2 drops
Vetiver 2 drops
Palmarosa 3 drops
30ml (1fl oz) bubble bath

Shower Gels

Sometimes a bath is just not practical. As an alternative, shower gels are a great way to give your body a quick treat – whether to boost your immune system or to ease stress-related eczema. An energising shower gel is better than caffeine for getting you going, and it refreshes and cleanses you too.

Shower gels can be a very gentle yet effective way of helping to treat a wide range of skin conditions. They can also be excellent for preventing insect bites and stings, and for reducing the itchiness, inflammation and infection that can accompany stings and sunburn. For this reason, shower gels are great for travelling. So if the mosquitoes line up to greet you when you arrive on holiday, try making the Gorgeous recipe, or create your own blend. I've had particularly good results using Vetiver, Lemongrass, Lavender, Cedarwood and Chamomile in various combinations. Don't try Lemongrass and German Chamomile together – they don't smell very nice!

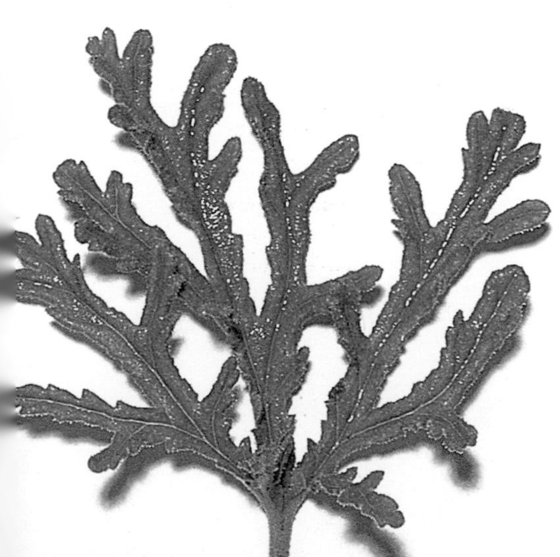

Gorgeous

As well as smelling wonderfully clean, clear and woody, this blend is excellent for stress-related skin conditions. Yarrow is a good anti-inflammatory oil, Sandalwood and Cedarwood are both great for acne-prone skins, and Bergamot is an immune stimulant and can help to clear infections. This recipe also makes a very effective insect repellant.

Yarrow 2 drops
Sandalwood 2 drops
Cedarwood 2 drops
Bergamot 4 drops
25ml (0.8fl oz) shower gel

Orange Peel Replacement Gel

Cellulite – that orange peel-like dimpling on hips, thighs and other body parts – can be reduced if you improve the circulation in affected areas. Rosemary is excellent for this, and it helps your body to cleanse and detoxify itself, as does Lemon. You should also drink lots of water – up to 2 litres (3.2 pints) a day. Geranium is useful if you indulge in a little chocolate worship, and if the thought of any kind of regime makes your heart sink. Its sweetness will lift your spirits and reduce cravings to a manageable level. It will also add a pleasant smell to the blend.

Rosemary 4 drops
Lemon 3 drops
Geranium 1 drop
20ml (0.6fl oz) shower gel

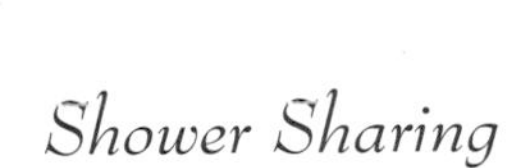

Shower Sharing

The generous of heart might choose to share this shower gel with someone special. The blend of oils encourages feelings of warmth and love – unless you like it so much that you want to keep it to yourself! It is a very potent gel – not least because of the wide range of essential oils it contains.

Rose 1 drop
Neroli 3 drops
Coriander 2 drops
Rosewood 2 drops
Vetiver 2 drops
30ml (1fl oz) shower gel

Wake Up Call

You are feeling tired – the alarm went off too early – you are jaded and don't know how you are going to get through the day. Try this invigorating blend: Peppermint to wake you up and clear your head, Rosemary to keep you alert and to ease any muscular aches or pains, Lemon and Coriander to aid detoxification. This is especially good if you are suffering from a hangover.

Rosemary 2 drops
Peppermint 3 drops
Coriander 2 drops
Lemon 2 drops
25ml (0.8fl oz) shower gel

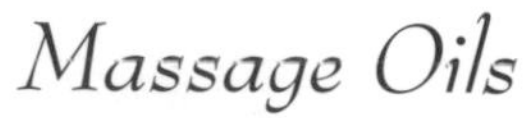

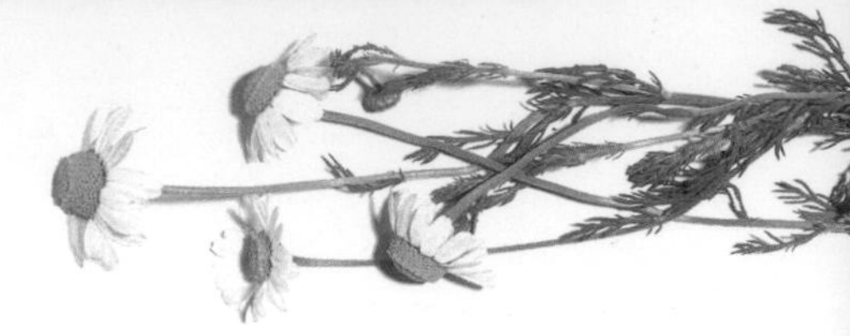

Massage Oils

Massage is one of the main ways of experiencing the benefits that essential oils offer, and you do not have to be a professional Aromatherapist to use them in this way. Any of the carrier oils can be used; I would suggest Grapeseed oil as it is relatively inexpensive and easy to obtain. Massage oils can also be used as intensive moisturisers for your skin, either by adding a spoonful of a blend to your bath or by applying the oil after bathing. Macadamia Nut oil is one of the more expensive carrier oils but it soaks into the skin relatively quickly and does not leave any residue. If you would like a high quality carrier oil that is not as expensive, Sweet Almond oil is a good alternative.

If your skin is very dry, try enriching your chosen carrier by adding 5ml (1 teaspoon) of Jojoba or Avocado oil to the recipe. This will give the final blend a silkier texture, and your skin will feel much softer.

Calendula can be a useful carrier oil if you are trying to reduce the effects of scar tissue or stretch marks. Some people find that it is absorbed extremely quickly into the skin, so if you have dry or combination skin, try blending it with Jojoba oil.

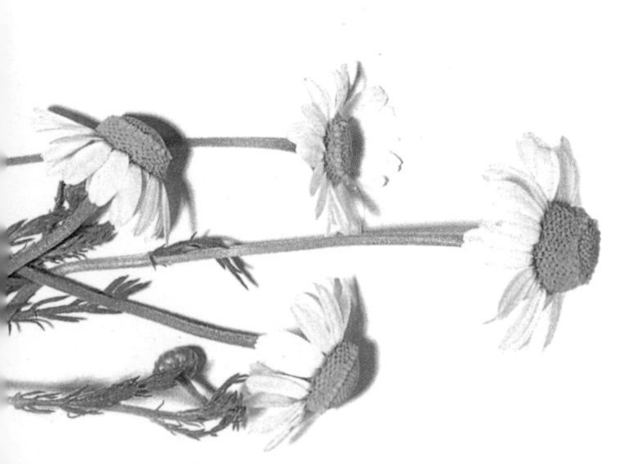

Anti-Stretch Marks

Try this blend to help remove stretch marks after giving birth. During pregnancy, plain Calendula oil can help prevent them.

Roman Chamomile 1 drop
Frankincense 2 drops
Lavender 1 drop
20ml (0.6fl oz) Calendula oil

Muscle Soother

If you have a stiff neck or tense shoulders, this blend will help to ease muscle spasm. It is warming and soothing, reducing any inflammation – and it will help to relieve pain.

German Chamomile 1 drop
Rosemary 2 drops
Lavender 2 drops
Marjoram 3 drops
20ml (0.6fl oz) Grapeseed oil

Poor Circulation

If you have poor circulation, this blend will warm your hands and feet – whatever the weather. Rosemary can also be used to improve circulation. Try using it in this blend instead of Vetiver.

Vetiver 2 drops
Ginger 3 drops
Grapefruit 3 drops
20ml (0.6fl oz) Grapeseed oil

Seduction

Treat this blend with care! It is very warming, soothing and cleansing. It smells like a tropical garden at night and is irresistible.

Patchouli 4 drops
Jasmine 3 drops
Lemon 3 drops
25ml (0.8fl oz) Grapeseed oil

Doze

This smoky, citrus-like blend is popular if you are having problems sleeping, either through overwork, aching muscles or stress. Gently relaxing and comforting, it will have you snoozing in no time.

Vetiver 3 drops
Lavender 4 drops
Orange 4 drops
30ml (1fl oz) Grapeseed oil

Breathe Easy

Here is a wonderful oil which will help respiration if are suffering from a chest infection, hay fever or asthma. It will also help to ease aches and pains associated with winter colds and flu, clearing catarrh and encouraging you to breathe more easily.

Cedarwood 3 drops
Frankincense 3 drops
Benzoin 2 drops
20ml (0.6fl oz) Grapeseed oil

Clearing Cobwebs

Clear the cobwebs away from your mind and body with this energising blend, which is excellent when you want to make decisions or if you need to motivate yourself. Lemongrass and Ginger are both excellent for muscular aches and pains, and together with Geranium, they help ease digestive difficulties. The overall effect is gently warming and tropical.

Ginger 3 drops
Lemongrass 2 drops
Geranium 3 drops
20ml (0.6fl oz) Grapeseed oil

Perfumes

Many of today's perfumers start by blending essential oils drop by drop until exactly the right fragrance is attained. However, many modern perfumes are subsequently produced under laboratory conditions, using chemically-derived constituents which mimic essential oils. I feel they are not nearly as good as the real thing. You may find, like me, that once you start blending essential oil perfumes, you will no longer want to use these commercially-produced products.

Most of the perfumes here contain more than three essential oils. For everyday wear, citrus or lighter-smelling oils are good. For evening wear you may like a heavier, muskier perfume which can be achieved by using more base notes – the woods and the roots.

When trying out the recipes, it is advisable to shake the perfume well after you have blended the oils, so that they mix well with the surgical spirit or alcohol. Allow the blend to settle for two days before using it.

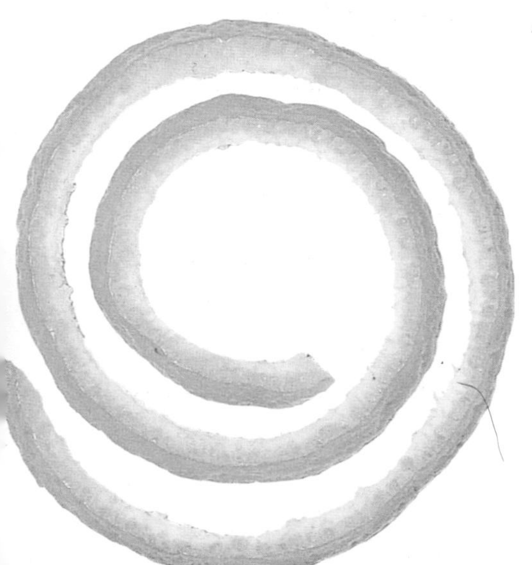

Citrus Grove

An excellent blend for daytime use. The Grapefruit and Lemon make this perfume light and fresh.

Grapefruit 4 drops
Lemon 3 drops
Patchouli 2 drops
Coriander 3 drops
40ml (1.3fl oz) surgical spirit or vodka
40ml (1.3fl oz) Rose Water or Orange Blossom Water

Tropical Nights

This beautiful blend has the exotic aroma of hot summer nights in the Orient, with the sweet-smelling Jasmine in bloom and the scent of Lemongrass in the air.

Jasmine 4 drops
Vetiver 2 drops
Lemongrass 2 drops
Patchouli 2 drops
Rose 2 drops
40ml (1.3fl oz) surgical spirit or vodka
40ml (1.3fl oz) Orange Blossom Water

Sanctity

A soothing yet subtle perfume with Rose, which really lifts the spirits, and Frankincense, which soothes and calms.

Rose 3 drops
Neroli 2 drops
Grapefruit 3 drops
Vetiver 2 drops
Frankincense 3 drops
40ml (1.3fl oz) surgical spirit or vodka
40ml (1.3fl oz) Rose Water

Forest

The whole forest in a bottle – roots, bark, fruits and flowers. This is a lovely woody, floral blend designed to improve your appetite for life.

Vetiver 4 drops
Rosewood 3 drops
Bergamot 2 drops
Grapefruit 2 drops
Jasmine 2 drops
40ml (1.3fl oz) surgical spirit or vodka
40ml (1.3fl oz) Rose Water or Orange Blossom Water

Head Turning

Who needs to go on a diet or have a face lift when you can create a perfume like this? It really will make heads turn!

Palmarosa 4 drops
Rosewood 5 drops
Lemongrass 2 drops
Jasmine 2 drops
40ml (1.3fl oz) surgical spirits or vodka
40ml (1.3fl oz) Rose Water

Young Love

Another light, fresh blend which is very soothing and calming. It is a wonderful perfume to wear when you are feeling anxious or insecure.

Cedarwood 6 drops
Orange 2 drops
Neroli 3 drops
Lavender 5 drops
40ml (1.3fl oz) surgical spirit or vodka
40ml (1.3fl oz) Rose Water or Orange Blossom Water

SOAPS

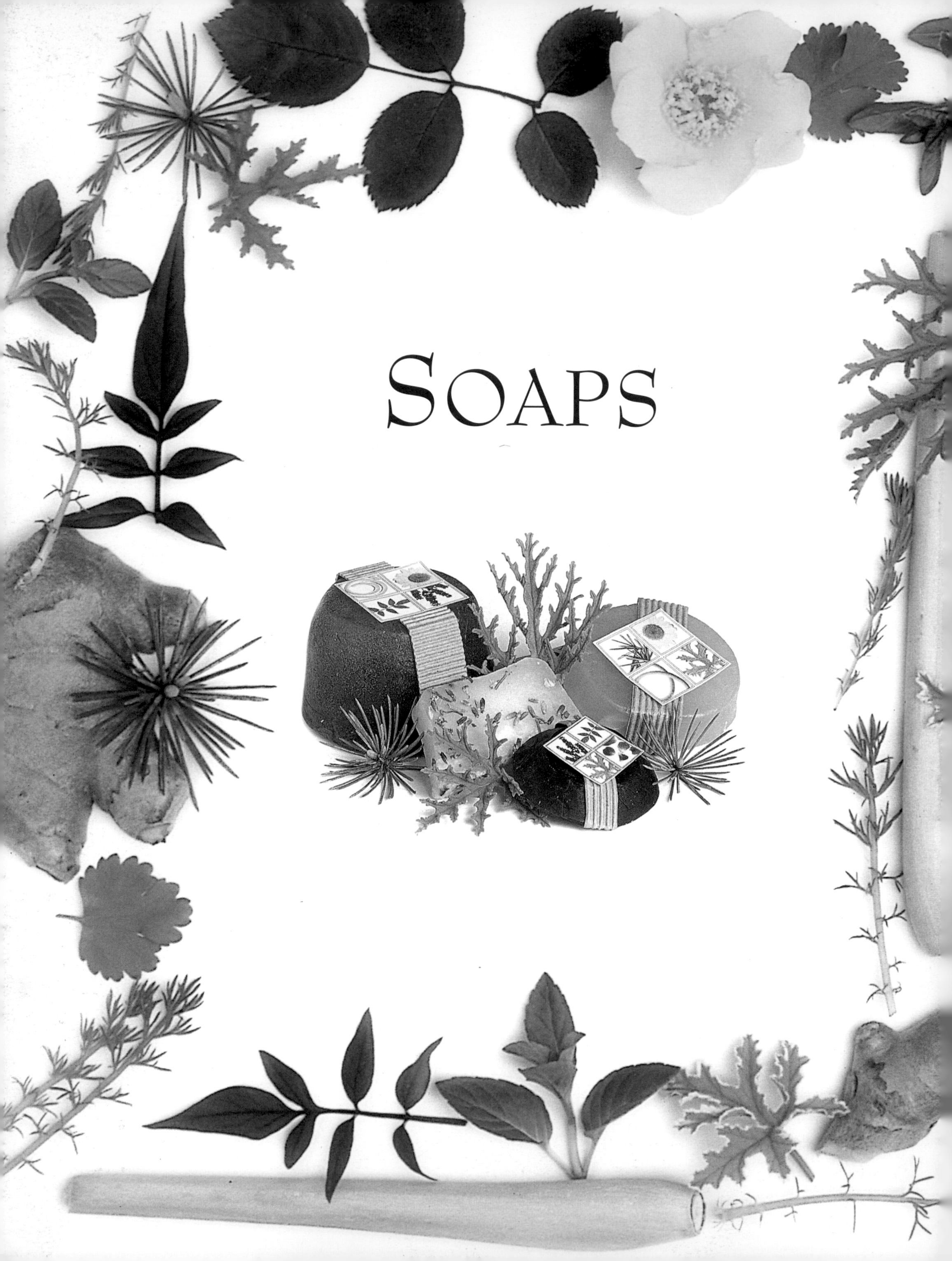

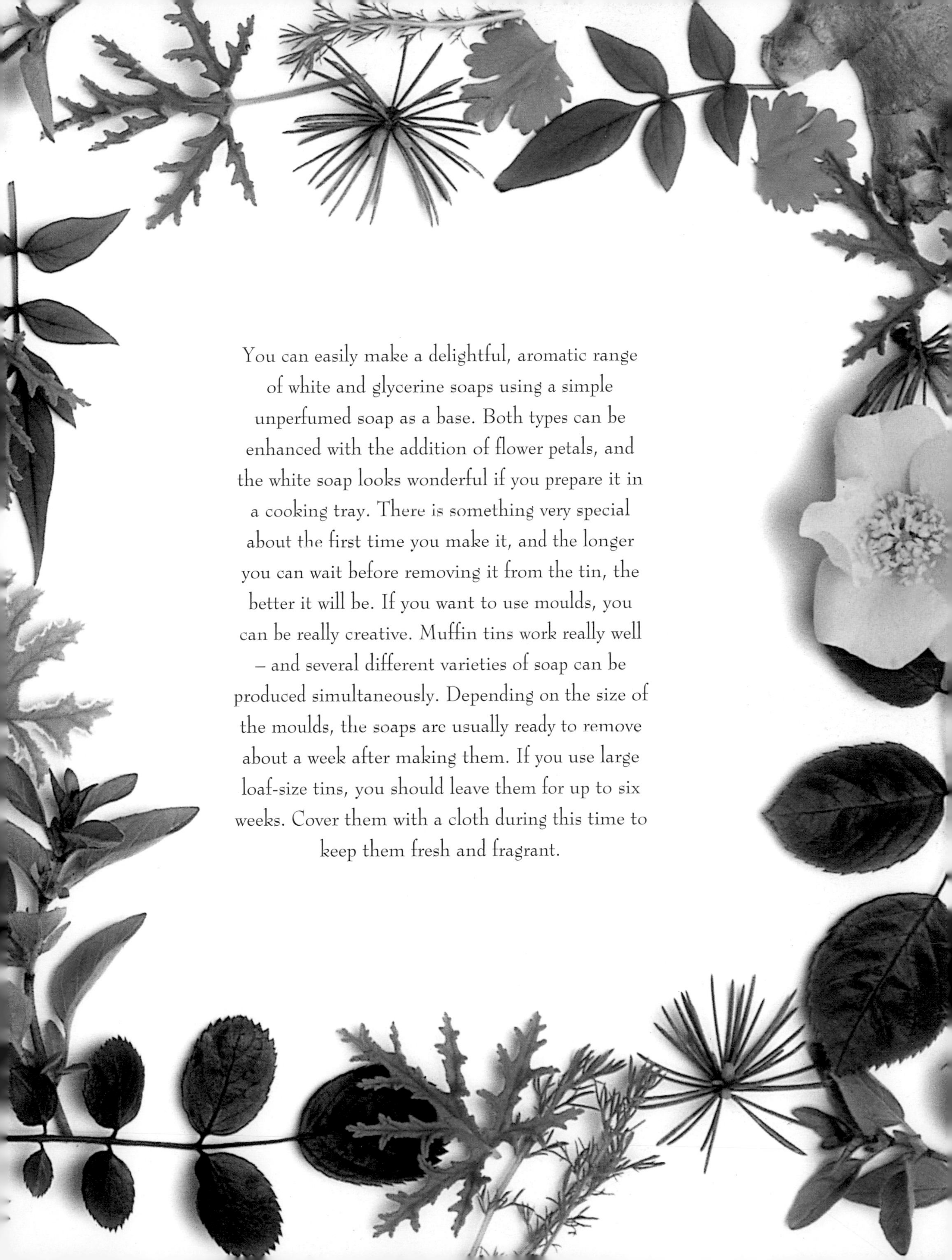

You can easily make a delightful, aromatic range of white and glycerine soaps using a simple unperfumed soap as a base. Both types can be enhanced with the addition of flower petals, and the white soap looks wonderful if you prepare it in a cooking tray. There is something very special about the first time you make it, and the longer you can wait before removing it from the tin, the better it will be. If you want to use moulds, you can be really creative. Muffin tins work really well – and several different varieties of soap can be produced simultaneously. Depending on the size of the moulds, the soaps are usually ready to remove about a week after making them. If you use large loaf-size tins, you should leave them for up to six weeks. Cover them with a cloth during this time to keep them fresh and fragrant.

Materials

Baking tray (or a shallow dish) This is excellent if you want to produce large batches of soap. A loaf tin could also be used.

Muffin tin This is the most useful item for soap-making. Round, fairly quick-drying soaps can be made in convenient sizes. Also, if things are planned carefully, the tin can be used to create a range of different soaps. Simply follow the first two soap-making steps (see pages 50–51), then decant the mixture into the muffin tin. Add the essential oils to each soap: in the shallow tin shown, 10 drops per 20ml (0.6fl oz) dish of the muffin tin. Stir thoroughly and allow to set.

Moulds Anything can be used as a mould: jelly moulds, plant pots, loaf tins or jars. Let your imagination run wild!

Grater The soap is grated with this. Grate it as finely as you can, so that it dissolves easily during the heating process.

Unscented soap Fragrance-free hypoallergenic soaps are an excellent base for the recipes in this chapter.

Glycerine Glycerine soap is considered much more beneficial for the skin than ordinary white soap. Glycerine is available from most good chemists.

Olive oil, Jojoba oil, Avocado oil and Sweet Almond oil These oils have good moisturising qualities and can be added to the recipes – especially if you are making soap for someone with dry skin.

Dried flowers Can be used to decorate or colour soap. They are available from health food shops and florists.

Measuring jug and spoons Liquid ingredients are measured in these.

Sharp knife Use this to cut and remove the soap after it has hardened in a baking tray.

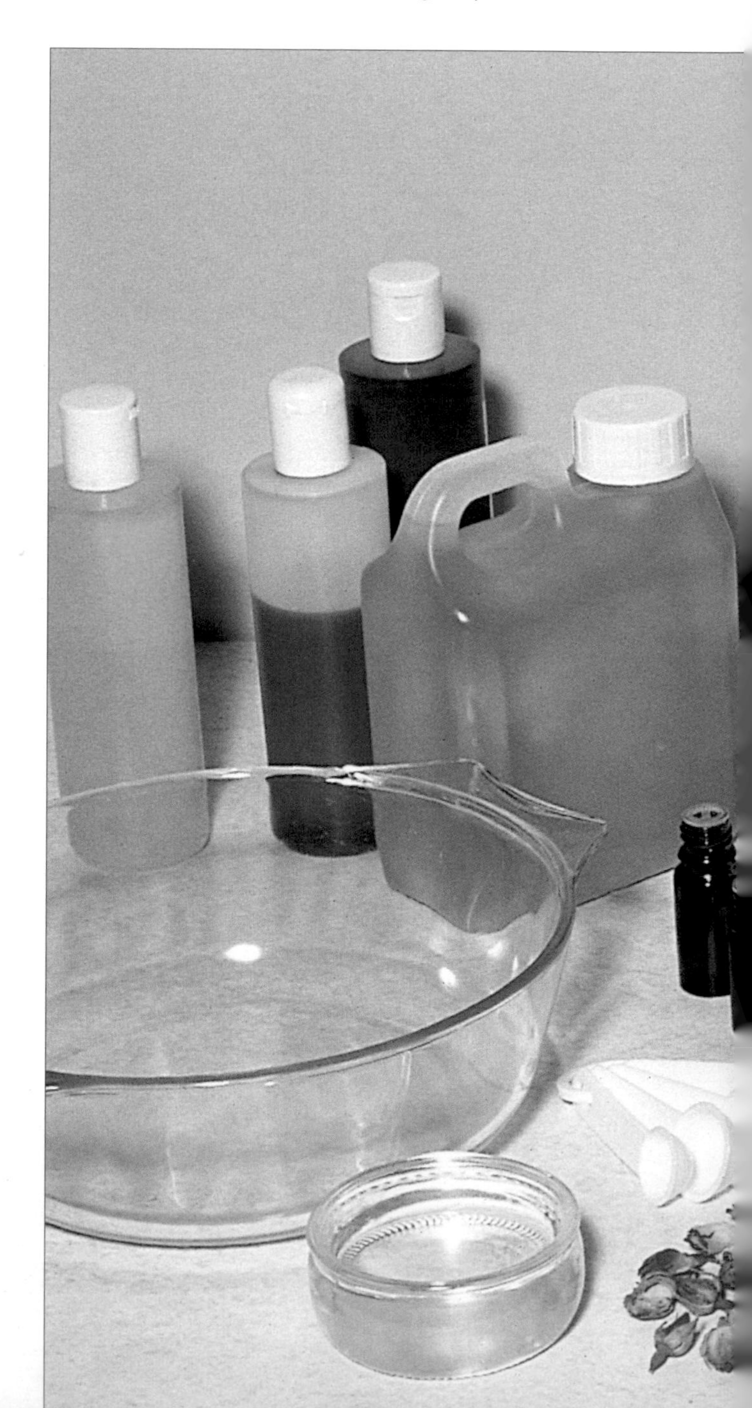

Metal spoon As the soap melts, it is blended with this. Do not use a wooden spoon, as it would be unhygienic and difficult to clean.

Greaseproof paper It is easier to remove soap from a mould if it is lined with greaseproof paper – and the soap is less likely to be damaged. Also, soap can be wrapped in greaseproof paper after it has been cut into bars, to keep the scent fresh.

Metal saucepan Water is heated in this.

Heat-resistant glass bowl Ingredients are mixed in this. It is also placed on top of the metal saucepan over hot water and soap is dissolved in it.

Essential oils See recipes.

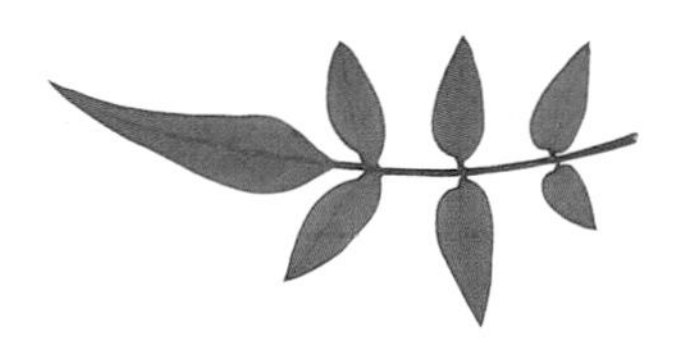

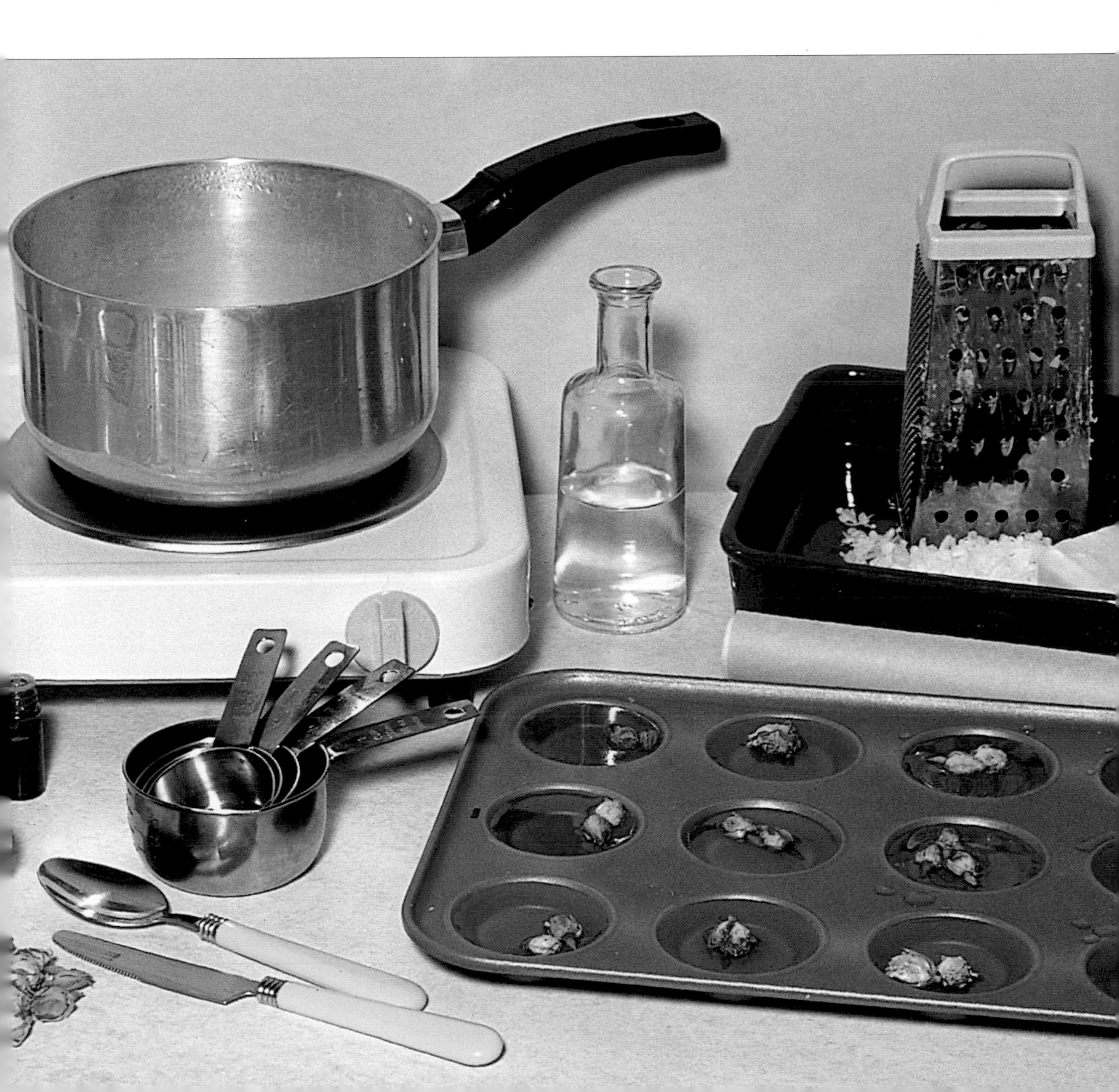

Techniques

Preparing white soap

A whole range of soaps can be made quickly and easily using the following method. The base used here is an unperfumed white soap which is heated. It can take a little time to melt, so be patient and persevere. Do not be tempted to turn up the heat to speed up the process, as a high heat can cause the soap to boil too fast and it will burn or 'curdle'.

The majority of essential oils will evaporate during the soap-making process – both when they are added to the warm mixture and while they are drying. To compensate for this, this technique uses up to 35 drops of essential oils per 50g (1.8oz) of base soap.

If you have dry skin, certain oils are beneficial and will act as moisturisers. I therefore usually add one of the following to the soap base: Olive oil, Jojoba oil, Avocado oil or Sweet Almond oil.

You will need

Grater ~ 300g (10.6oz) white soap
Glass bowl ~ Water
Measuring jug ~ Metal saucepan
Metal spoon
5 tablespoons Olive, Jojoba, Avocado or Sweet Almond oil
Essential oils
4 tablespoons of dried flower petals
Shallow dish ~ Knife
Greaseproof paper

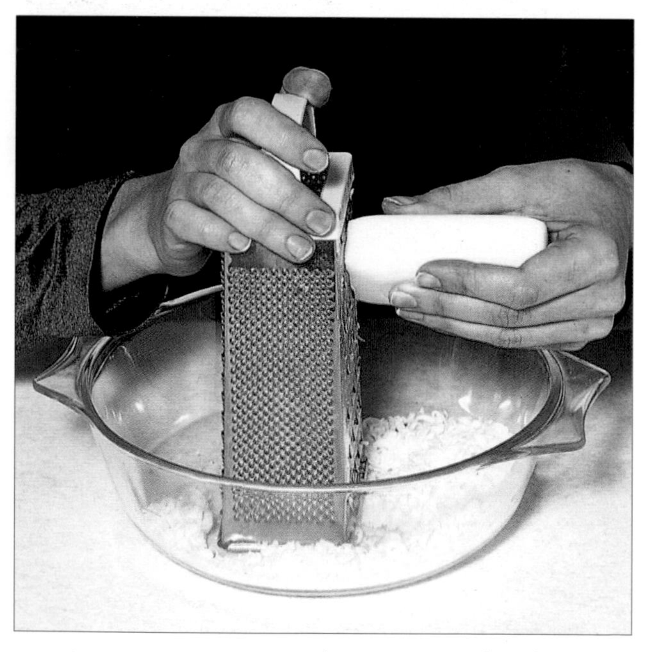

1. Grate 300g (10.6oz) of soap into a glass bowl.

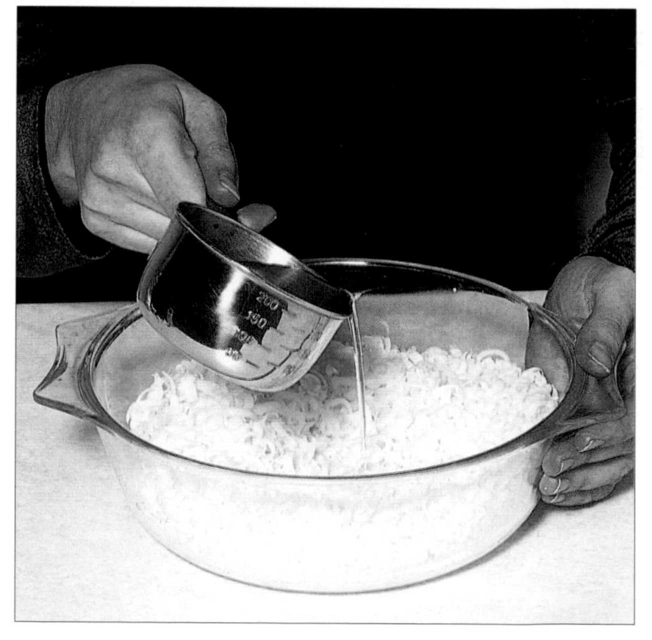

2. Measure 500ml (16fl oz) of water and pour it over the grated soap.

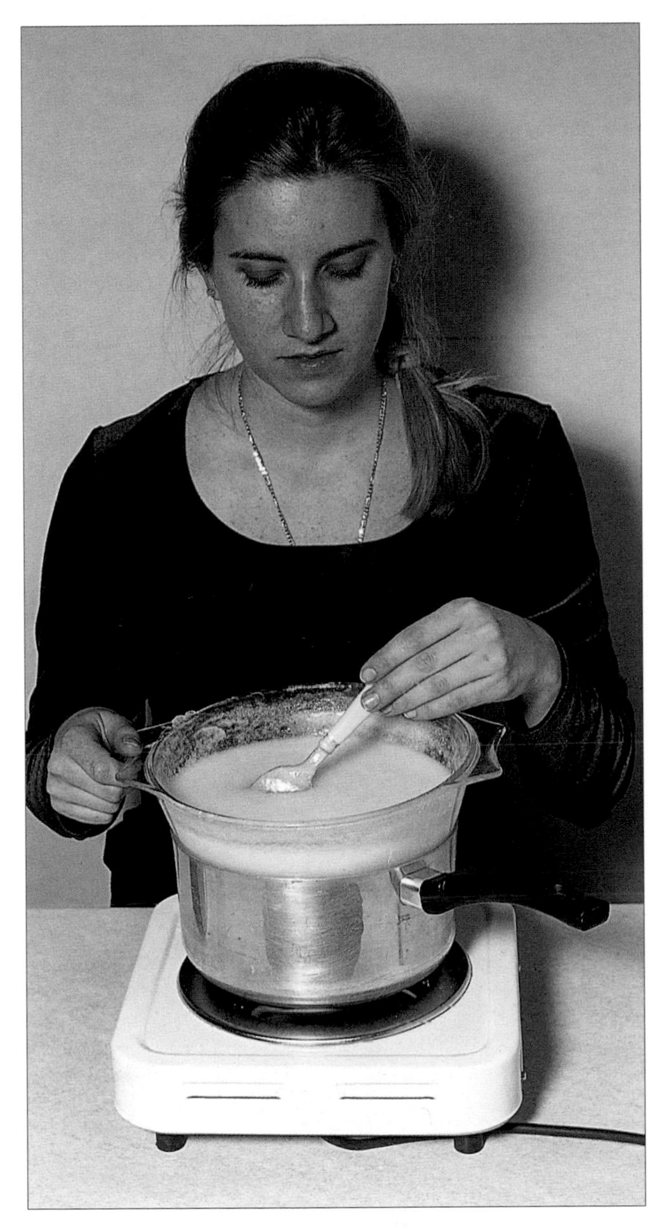

3. Place the bowl over a saucepan of boiling water. Heat gently for approximately 10 to 15 minutes, stirring continuously with a metal spoon, until the soap melts. Push out any lumps using the back of the spoon until the mixture is completely smooth. Remove from the heat.

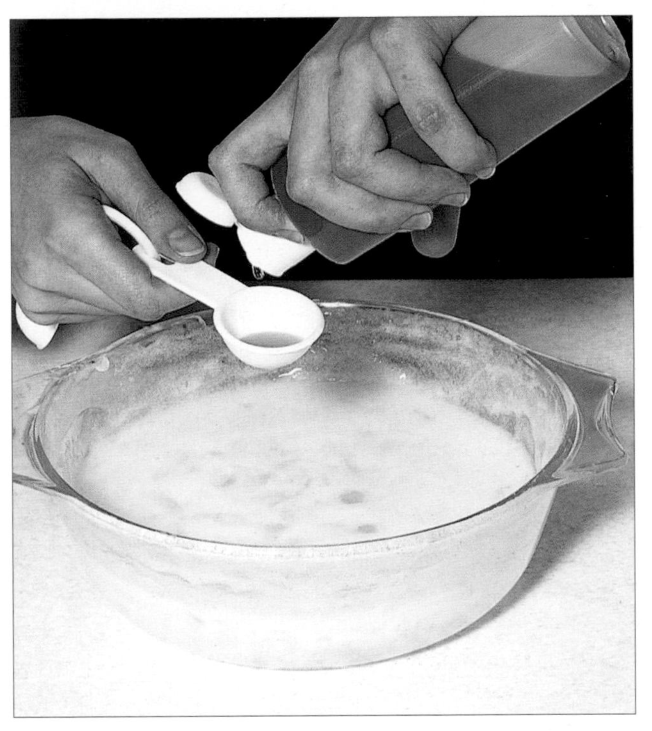

4. Add 5 tablespoons of Olive, Jojoba, Avocado or Sweet Almond oil to enrich the soap (optional).

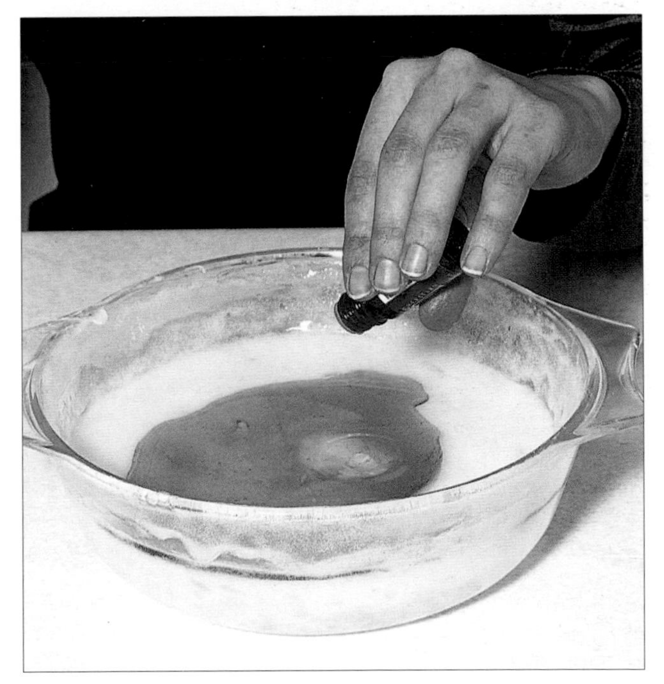

5. Add 200 drops of essential oils.

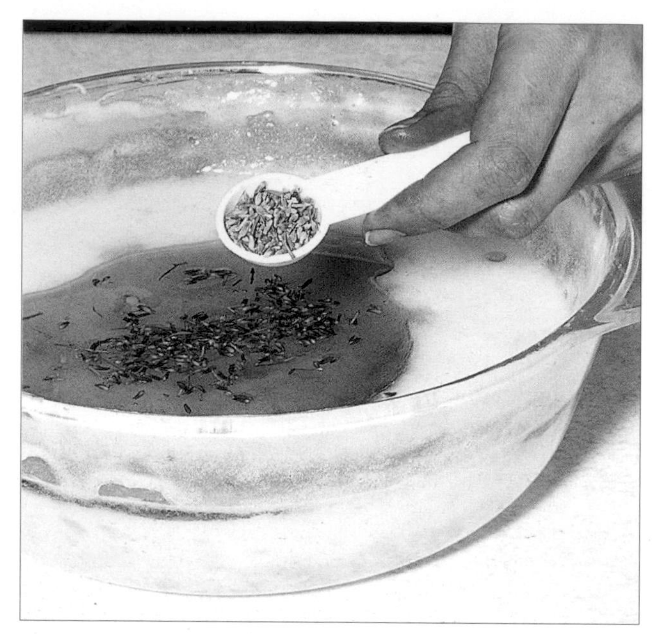

6. Add 4 tablespoons of dried flower petals to the mixture. For a different effect, you can add the dried flower petals at stage 8, after decanting.

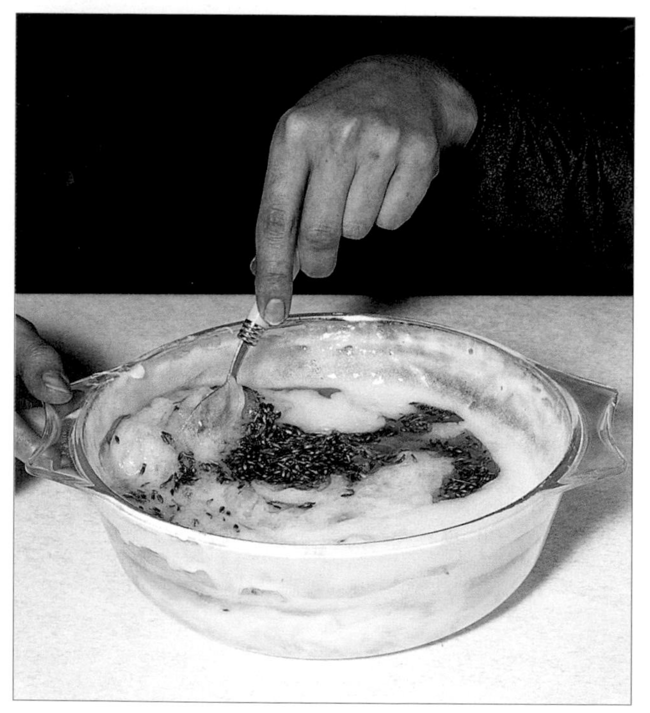

7. Mix the ingredients using a metal spoon.

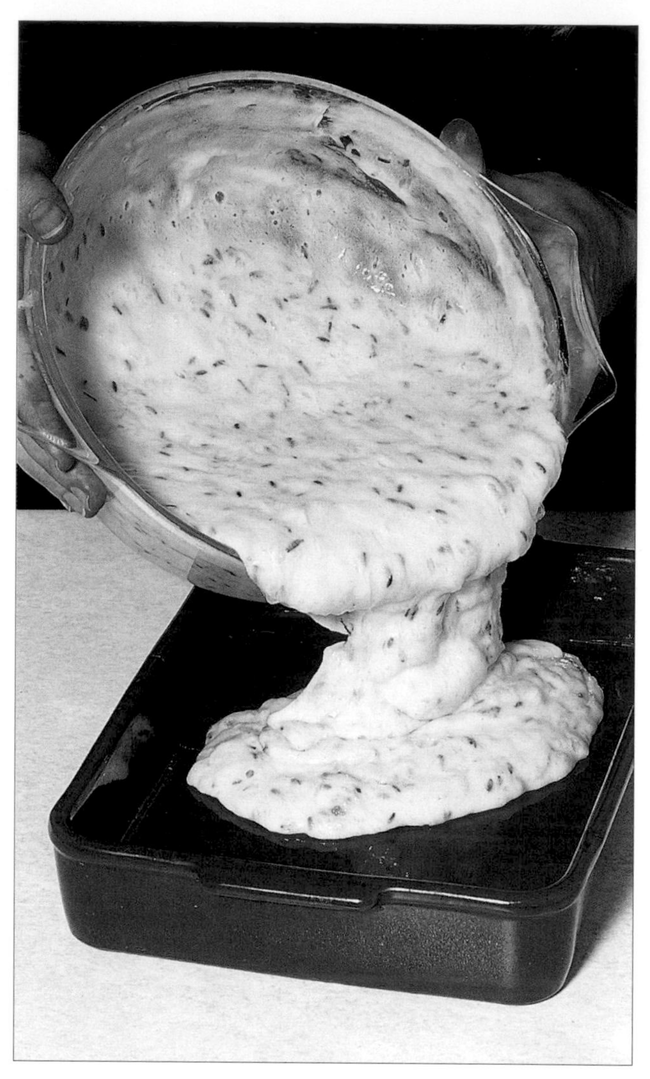

8. Decant the mixture into a shallow dish. Leave to cool and set until firm. This can take up to a week, depending on how fresh the base soap used is. If you are adding the flower petals at this stage, you can create some unusual effects by sprinkling them on as the blend is starting to set. Try sticking dried rosebuds in the top of the soap for a completely floral bathroom treat.

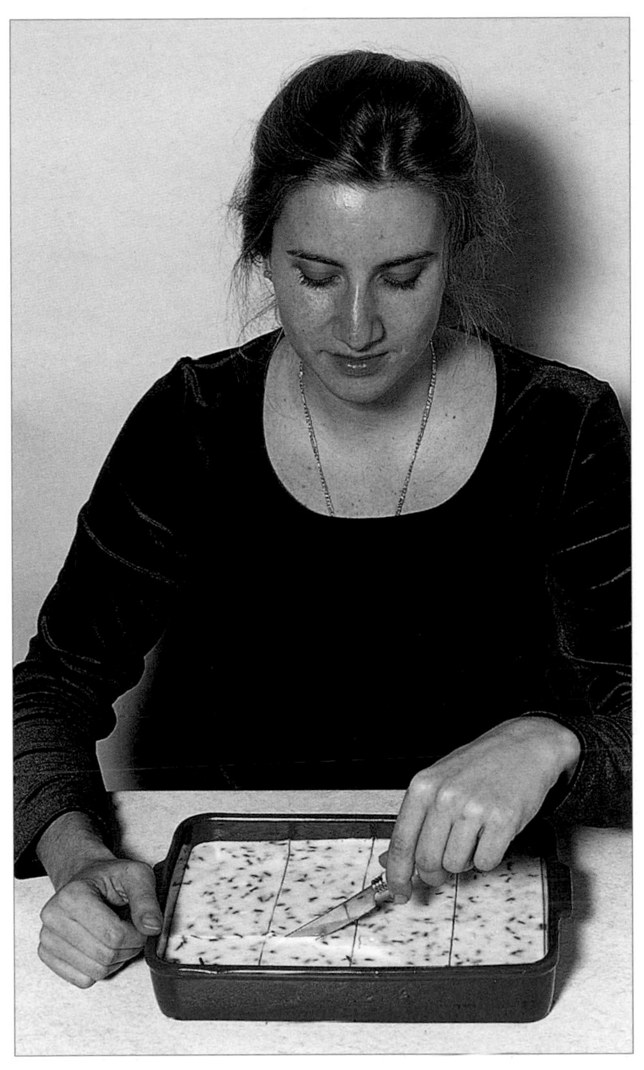

9. Divide the soap into squares using a knife.

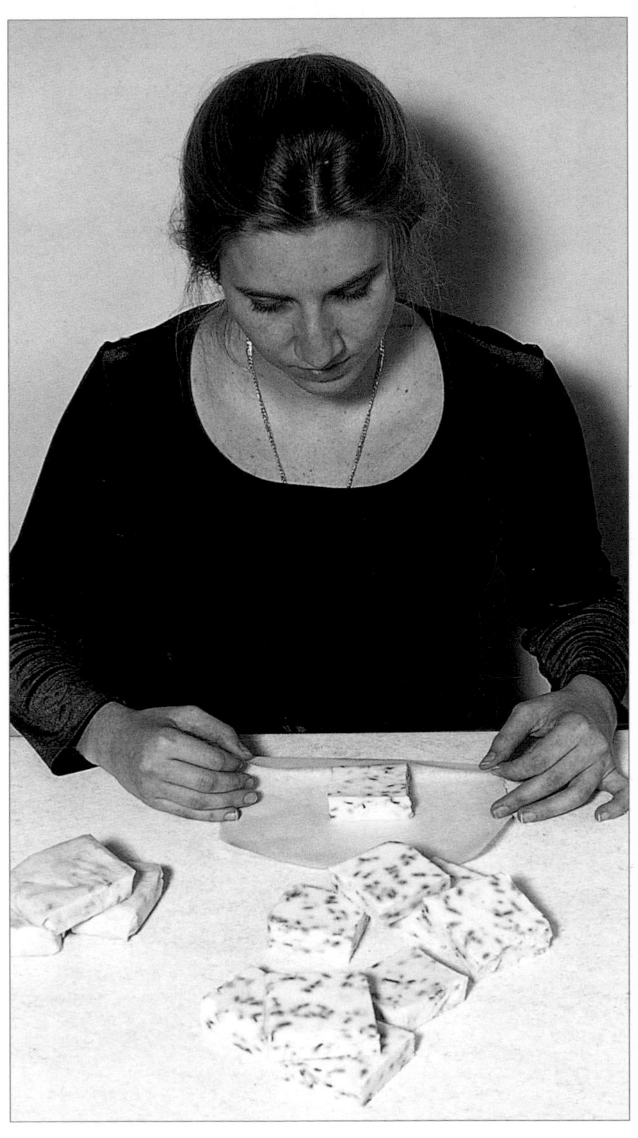

10. Remove the squares from the dish using a knife, then wrap them in greaseproof paper. Store in a cool place to dry thoroughly. This usually takes a couple of days.

Discolouration

Whenever you add flowers to soap, you should expect some discolouration as the soap dries. This is normal and does not affect the quality of the soap.

Preparing glycerine soaps

If you add glycerine to grated unperfumed soap and water, you will create a translucent soap. As with the white soap, some essential oils will act as colouring agents. I have chosen to use whole rosebuds in this demonstration, but any dried flower petals could be used.

Glycerine soaps are much more moist than white soaps, and it is better not to wrap them up, but to store them on a plate so they can dry until firm to touch.

You will need

Glass bowl ~ Measuring jug
Flower water
500ml (16fl oz) glycerine
Half a bar – 80g (2.8oz) – of white soap
Grater ~ Saucepan
Metal spoon
56 drops essential oil(s)
Dried flowers ~ Baking tray

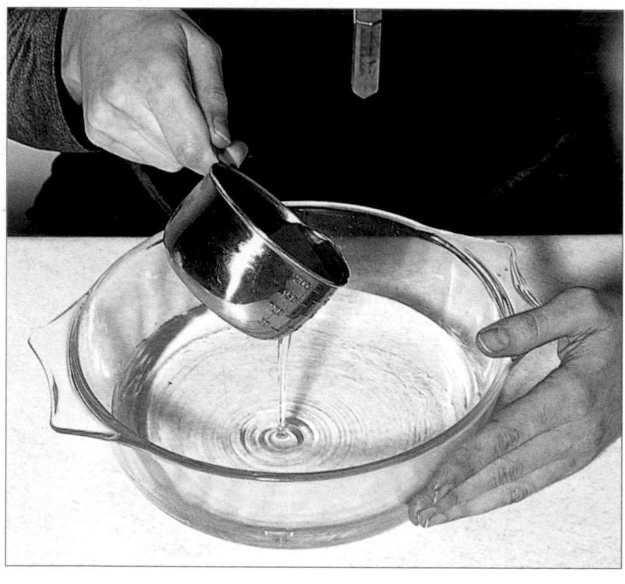

1. Pour 500ml (16fl oz) of flower water into a glass bowl. Add 500ml (16fl oz) of glycerine and half a bar of grated white soap.

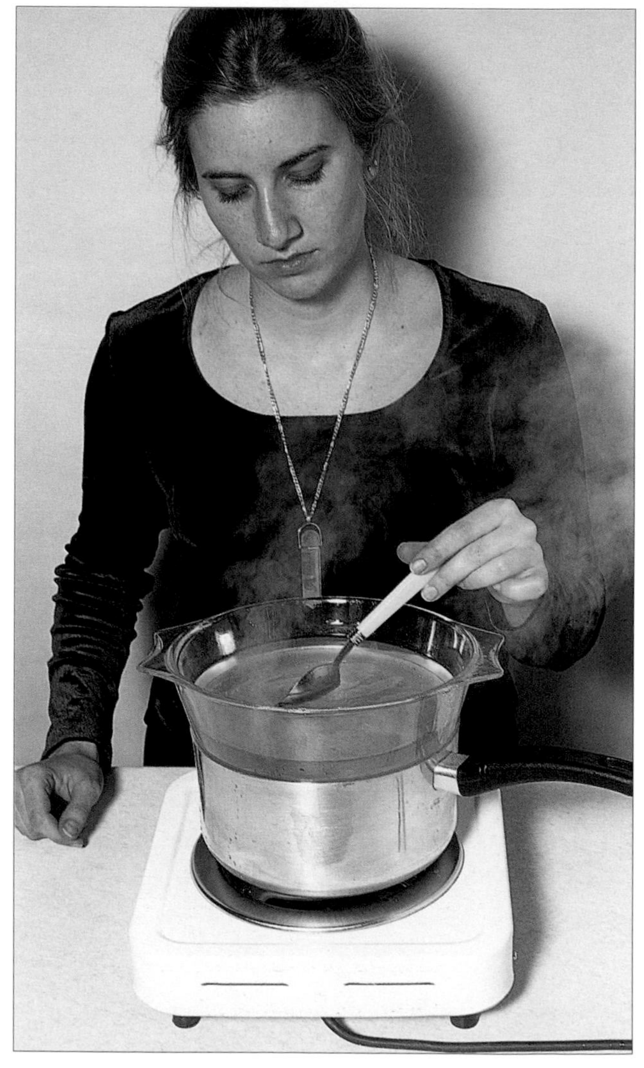

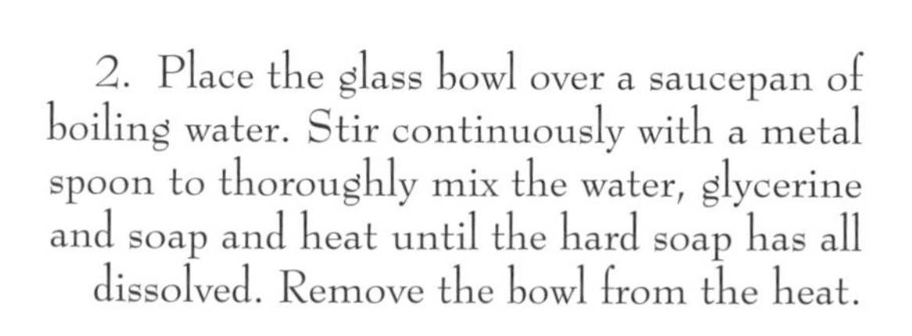

2. Place the glass bowl over a saucepan of boiling water. Stir continuously with a metal spoon to thoroughly mix the water, glycerine and soap and heat until the hard soap has all dissolved. Remove the bowl from the heat.

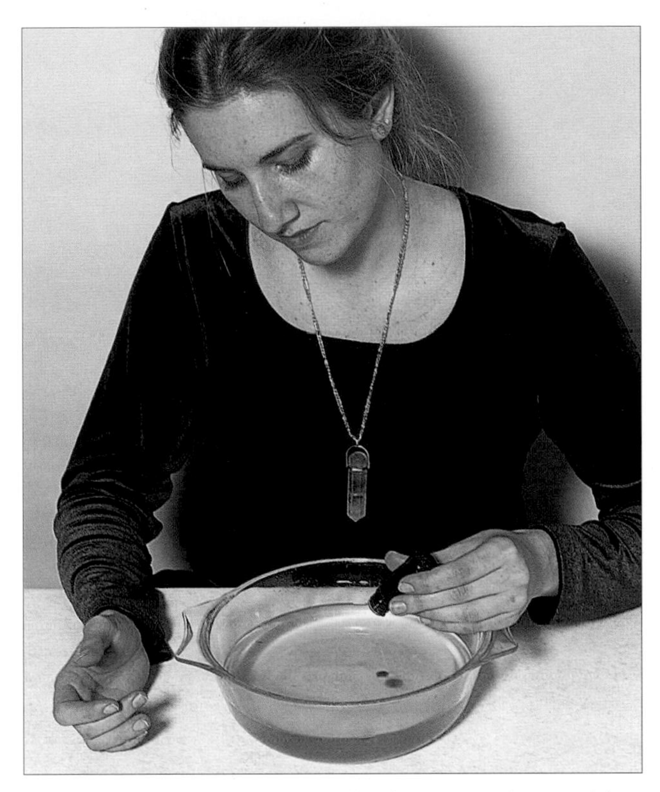

3. Add 56 drops of essential oil(s). Mix thoroughly. If you are making several kinds of soap at once, then instead of adding the essential oils at this stage, place a total of 6 drops in each muffin dish.

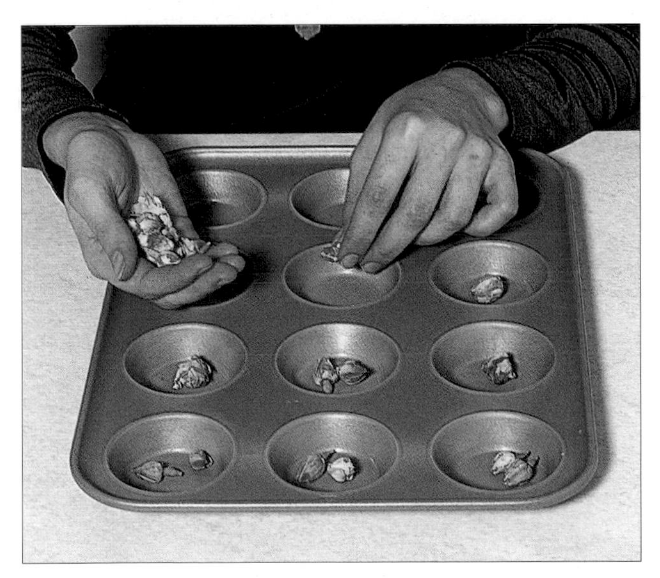

4. Lay a few rosebuds or flower petals in each dish of a muffin tin.

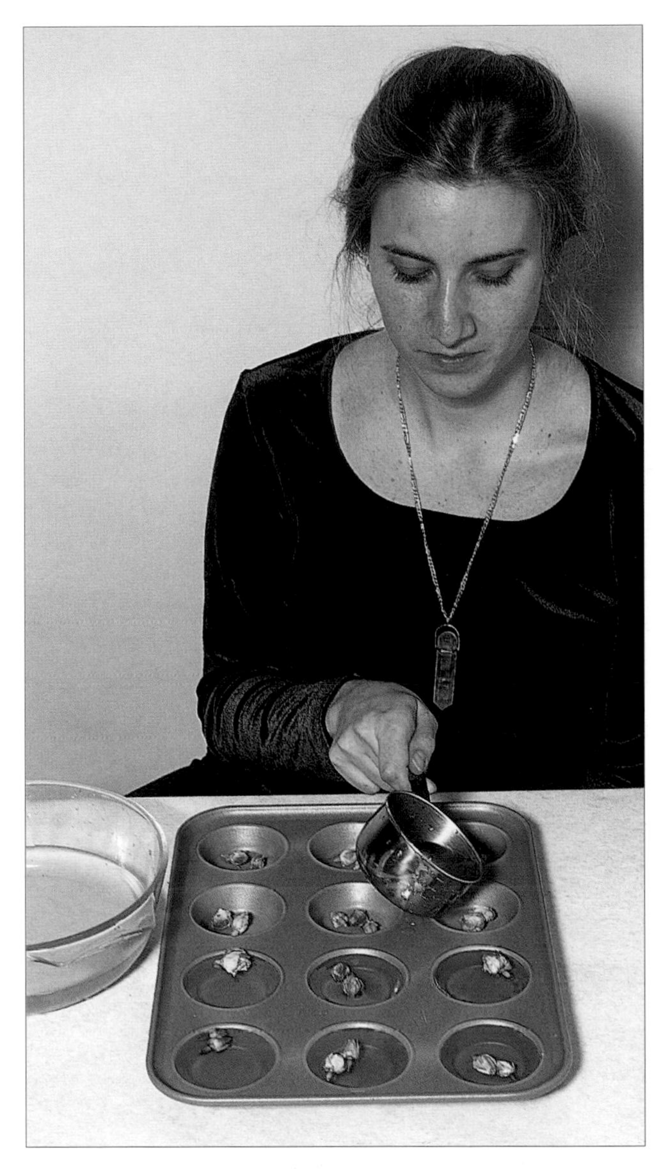

5. Ladle the soap mixture over the flowers/petals. Allow to set in a cool place for at least 48 hours.

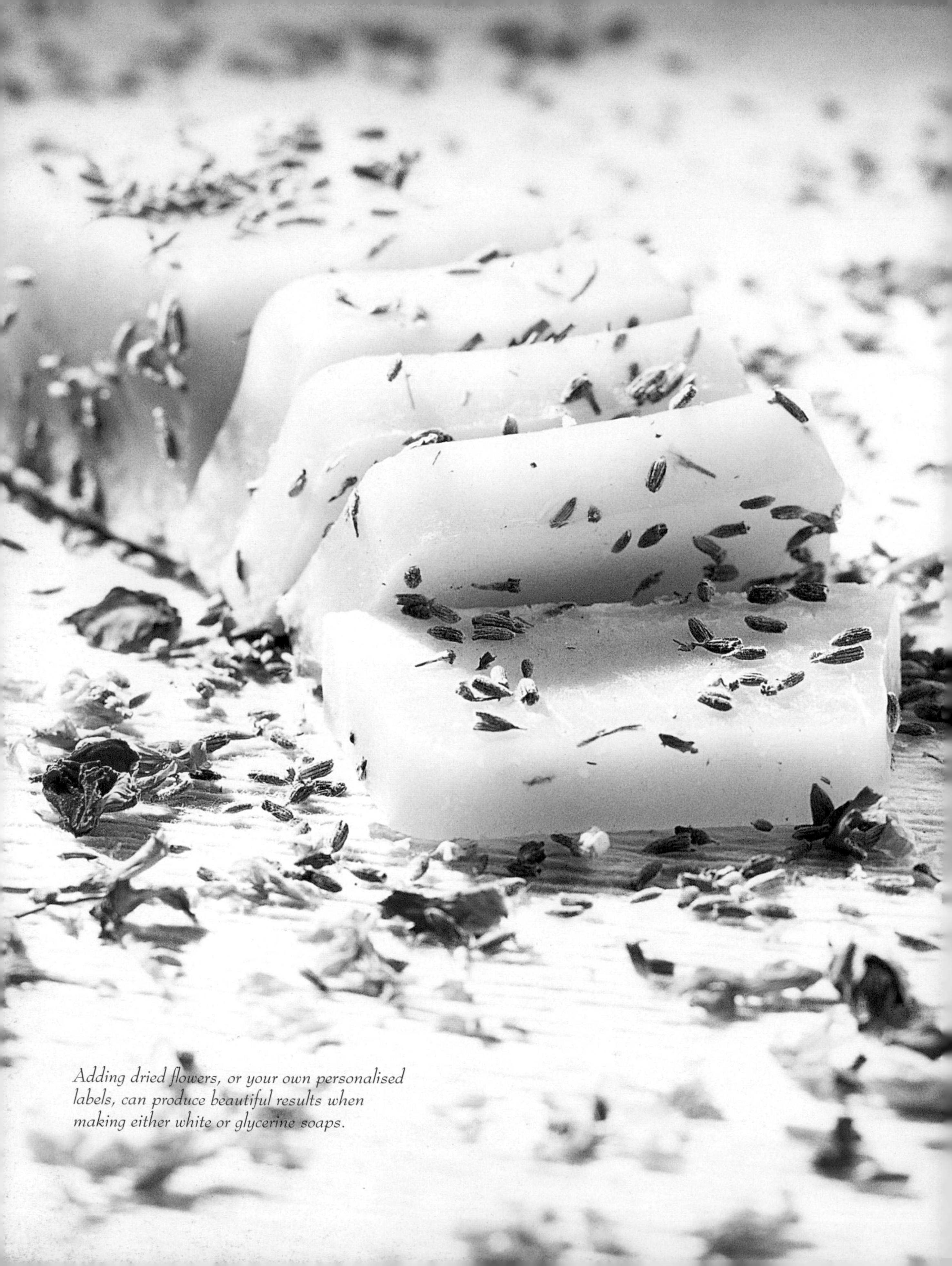

Adding dried flowers, or your own personalised labels, can produce beautiful results when making either white or glycerine soaps.

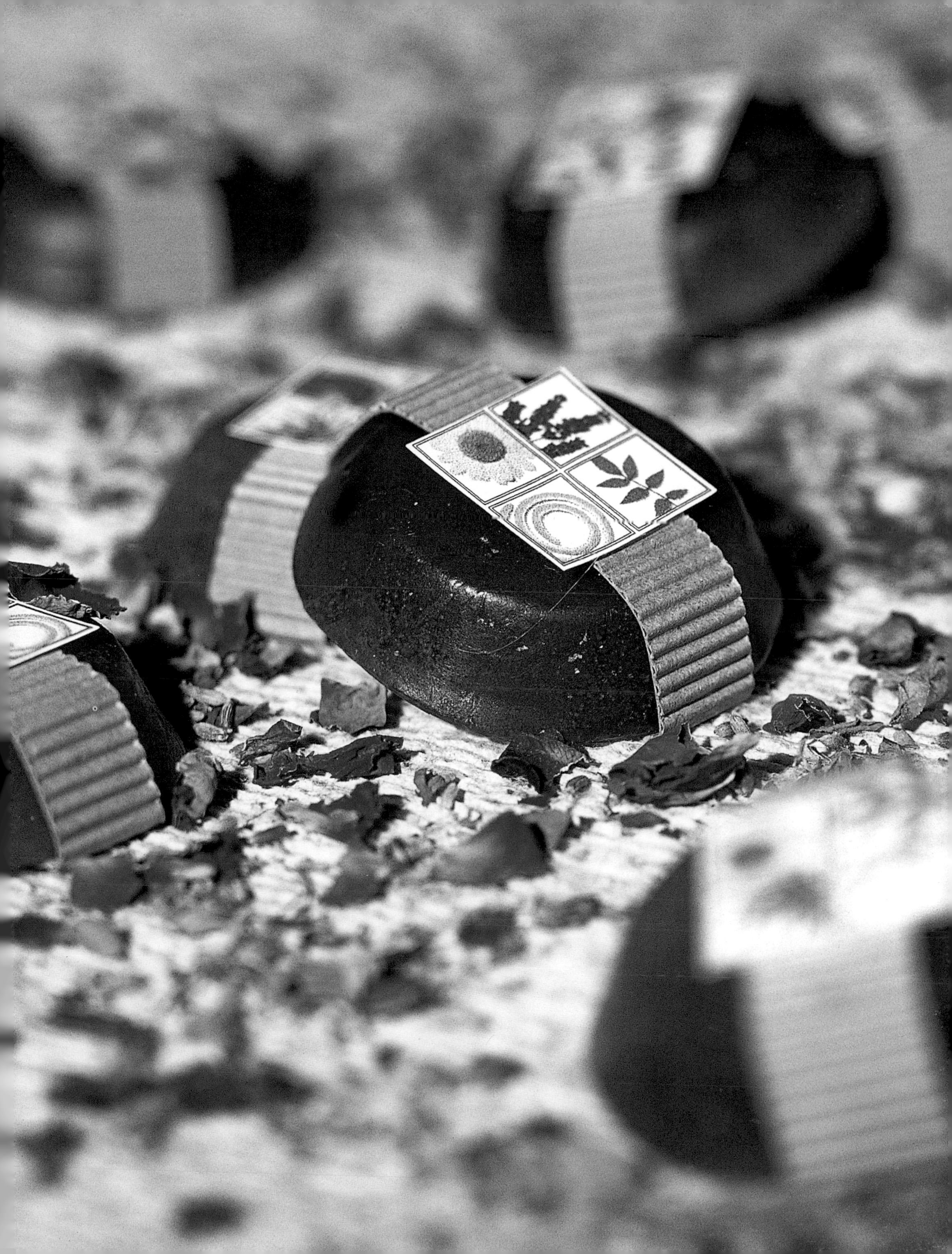

Colouring the soap

When you start decorating your soaps with different dried flowers, you are only one step away from adding colour. A simple flower water is an excellent colourant and it is simple enough to make your own. Simply put two to four heaped tablespoons of dried flowers in a mug, pour on 200ml (6.4fl oz) of boiling water and steep for five minutes. Strain off the liquid and use it instead of water at Step 2. The more flowers used, the stronger the colour produced. Try jasmine for a bright yellow, chamomile for pale greenish-yellow, rosebuds for pale pink, rosehips for a deep red, red rose petals for a claret brown (as shown here) and lavender for a greeny-brown.

There may be some discolouration later on if you include plant materials in a soap, but this is normal. The quality of the soap will not be affected.

Certain essential oils colour effectively if they are used in relatively high quantities. Vetiver and Benzoin will brown the soaps and Rose Absolute will redden them. Yarrow and German Chamomile will give a blue hue, which looks best in the glycerine soaps.

Carrier oils can also be used to add colour. Olive green, dark green, orange or yellow-brown can be achieved if you use Olive oil, Avocado oil, Calendula or Jojoba respectively. These oils also enrich the soaps, making them more effective as moisturisers.

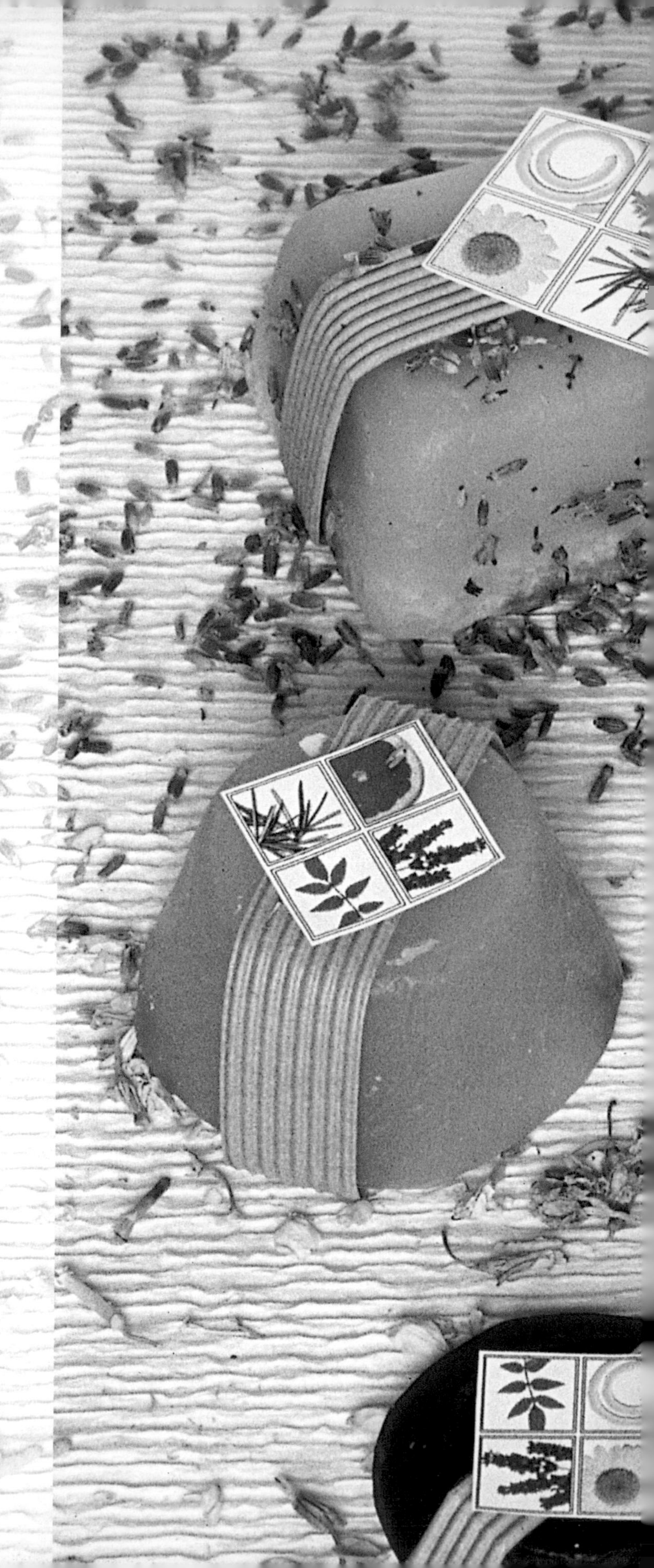

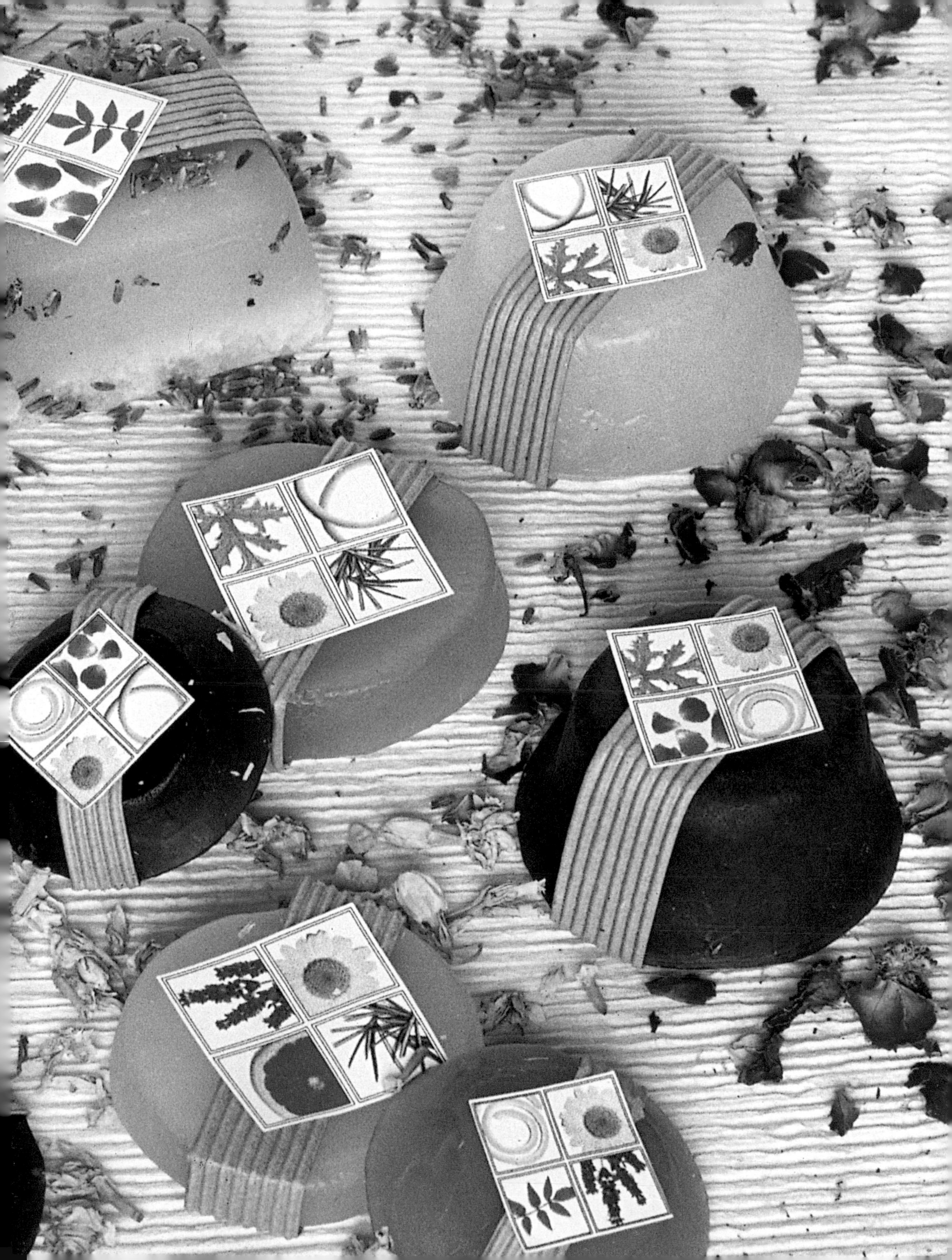

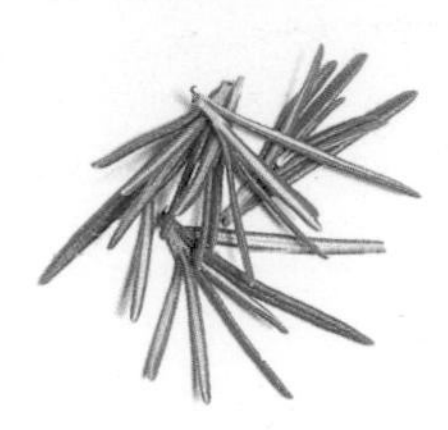

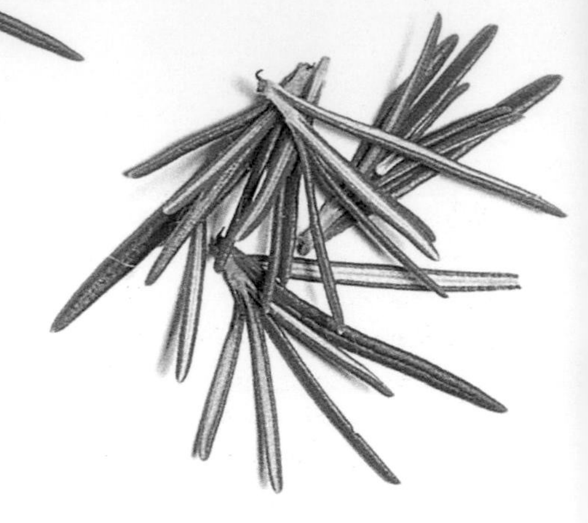

Recipes

White soaps

White soaps are the easiest ones to make as they involve no other ingredients apart from grated soap, water, essential oils (plus optional dried flowers and carrier oils).

The following recipes give you the amounts of essential oils to add to 30ml (1fl oz) of your liquid home-made soap mixture. This is the amount of soap you would put in one dish of a deep-dish muffin tin (also called an American muffin tin). This allows you to create different recipes in individual dishes of one muffin tin. Simply follow steps 1–4 of the technique shown on pages 46–49. Miss out step 5, but at step 8, pour the liquid soap into a muffin tin. Now you can add the essential oils to individual dishes, according to the recipes.

If you want to make one large batch of soap in a single container, as shown on pages 46–49, use the same recipes but multiply the numbers of drops by 6. This produces a slightly weaker mix, but makes for an easy conversion!

No Regrets

This is one for the morning after – for anyone who feels terribly guilty about having a good time and wants to scrub their conscience as well as their skin. A deep-cleansing blend with essential oils known for their soothing effects on the digestive system and their clearing effects on the mind.

Peppermint 4 drops
German Chamomile 2 drops
Grapefruit 5 drops
Rosemary 3 drops
30ml (1fl oz) of liquid home-made soap

Breathe Easier

A blend for those who suffer from upper respiratory tract infections and/or asthma. This is not going to help during an asthma attack, but it does help to reduce infection, makes it easier to breathe more deeply, helps reduce anxiety and can reduce the amount of associated catarrh.

Cedarwood 4 drops
Roman Chamomile 3 drops
Coriander 4 drops
Orange 4 drops
30ml (1fl oz) of liquid home-made soap

Chest Release

Beyond the ready-made Rosemary- or Eucalyptus-laden products for chest infections, there is room for something like this blend. These soothing, calming essential oils reduce coughing, boost the immune system, relieve the feeling of tightness in the chest and gently encourage sleep. Great for bronchitis in particular.

Lemon 4 drops
Yarrow 4 drops
Benzoin 3 drops
Marjoram 3 drops
30ml (1fl oz) of liquid home-made soap

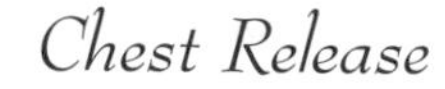

Skin Smoother

A lovely blend designed to encourage skin to return to its healthy state. Excellent for dry, cracked skin or acne, this is also a lovely soap to use if your skin is affected by your menstrual cycle.

Rose 4 drops
Benzoin 6 drops
Rosewood 4 drops
30ml (1fl oz) of liquid home-made soap

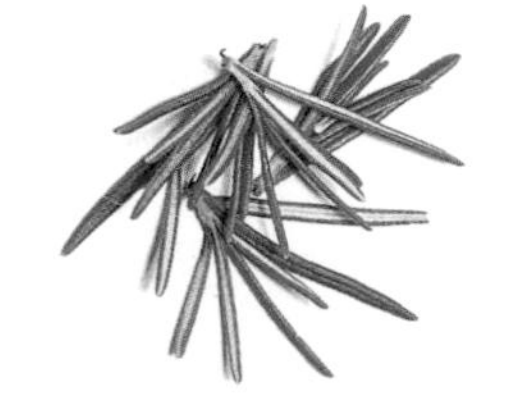

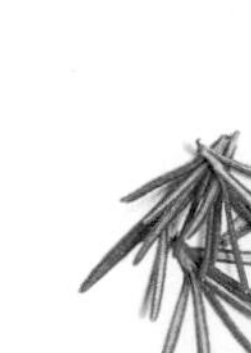

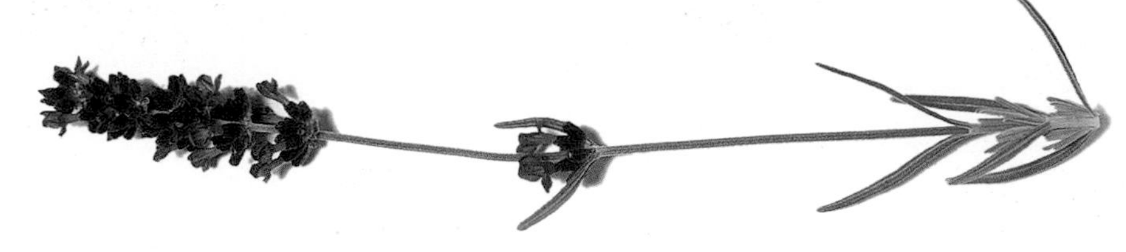

Recharge

When you tend to catch every bug going around, or your immune system seems to be on vacation, try this blend. Its gentle ingredients all help to recharge your batteries, fight off viruses and lift the sense of depression which can accompany long bouts of illness. Ginger also helps to warm aching muscles and joints.

Coriander 4 drops
Grapefruit 5 drops
Ginger 3 drops
Rose 4 drops
30ml (1fl oz) of liquid home-made soap

Winter Warmer

An extremely warming, yet gentle blend which boosts the immune system, helps to loosen catarrh and allows coughs to become less frequent and more productive. Ginger also helps to warm aching muscles and joints.

Benzoin 6 drops
Ginger 4 drops
Grapefruit 5 drops
30ml (1fl oz) of liquid home-made soap

Night Fever

Not just for use in the evenings, this blend helps to fight infections, boost your immune system, cool the body down and help restore you to good health. Also very useful if you are aware of feeling angry, if you have 'butterflies' in your stomach and/or pelvic infections.

Palmarosa 6 drops
Rosewood 5 drops
Peppermint 4 drops
30ml (1fl oz) of liquid home-made soap

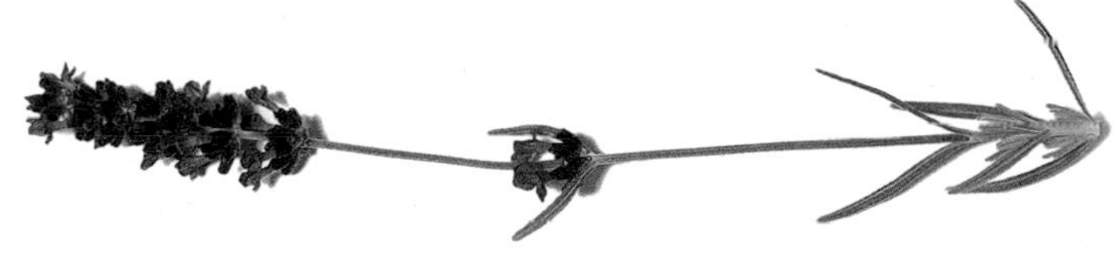

No Restrictions

This is great for those recovering from acute respiratory conditions where the chest feels constricted, there's quite a bit of catarrh, a feeling of fuzzy-headedness and a lot of lethargy. Imagine you are walking through the forest and you suddenly enter a patch of sunwarmed air, redolent with the smell of hot pine or cedarwood. This blend will make you breathe deeper, clear your nasal passages and remind you of what it feels like to have the energy to get up and get well again.

Cedarwood 4 drops
Rosemary 4 drops
Lavender 4 drops
Orange 4 drops
30ml (1fl oz) of liquid home-made soap

Letting Go

For those who suffer from constipation, this blend soothes uncomfortable spasms, bloating and build-up in the gut, making it easier to pass stools painlessly. Incidentally, it's also rather good if you are worrying unduly about something and finding it hard to let go of an idea or a way of life.

Peppermint 4 drops
Marjoram 4 drops
Orange 6 drops
30ml (1fl oz) of liquid home-made soap

Clearing Cobwebs

This is extremely useful for clearing catarrh and helping reduce the pain and swelling of sinusitis. It will leave your head feeling clearer and less constricted.

Lemon 3 drops
Coriander 6 drops
Rosemary 2 drops
Yarrow 4 drops
30ml (1fl oz) of liquid home-made soap

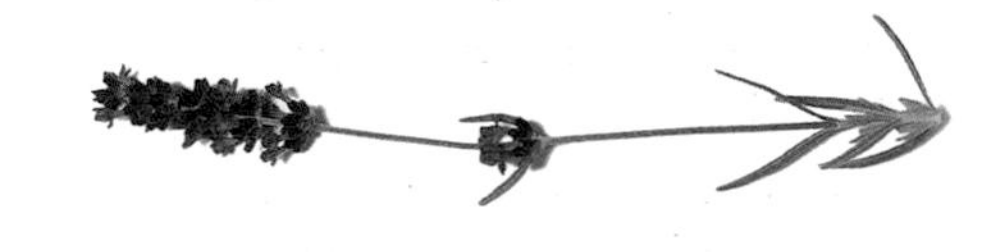

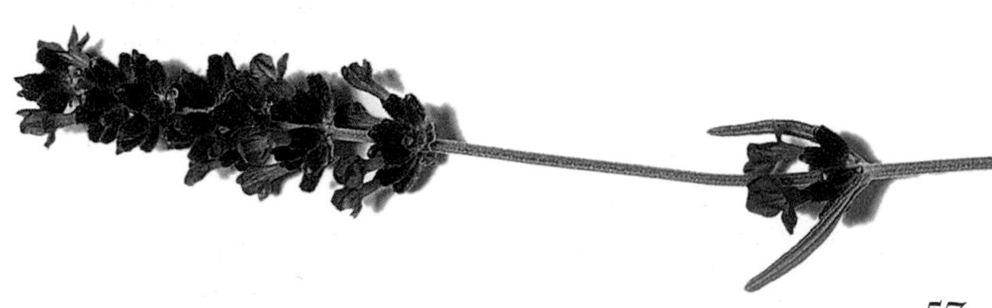

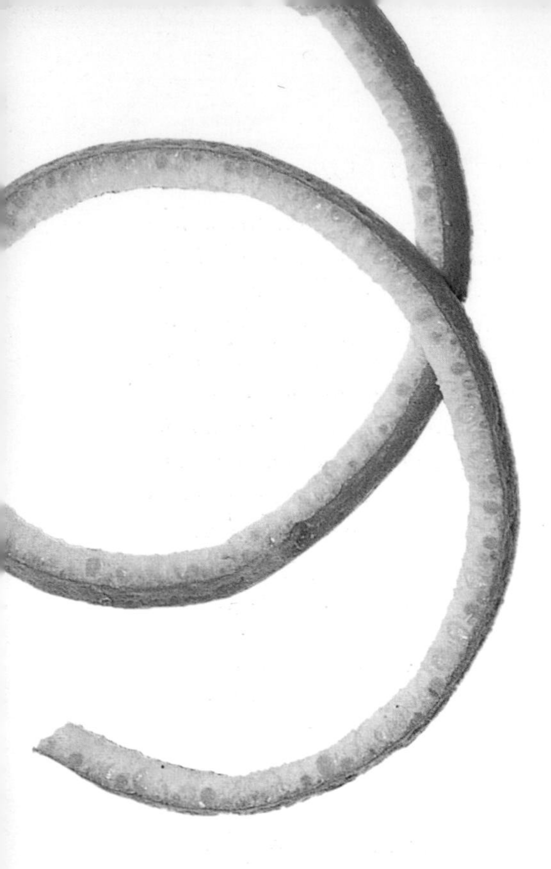

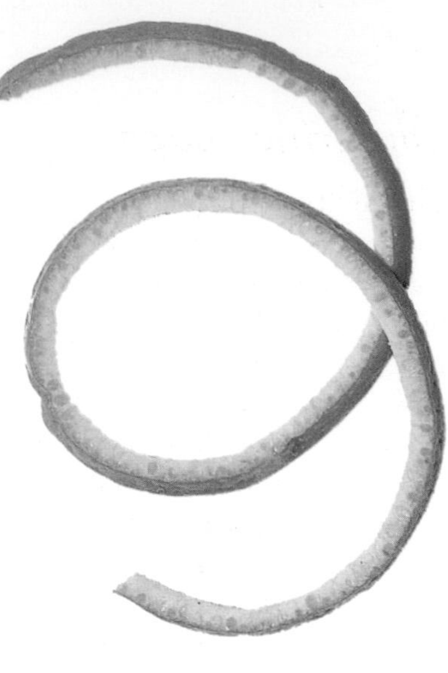

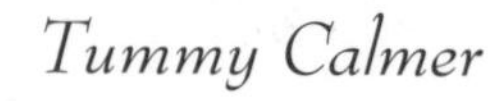

Tummy Calmer

Ideal for an inflamed gut, or when great pain is felt in the bowels, this soothing, cooling blend reduces inflammation, calms spasms and leaves you feeling a lot better.

Yarrow 5 drops
Peppermint 3 drops
Roman Chamomile 8 drops
30ml (1fl oz) of liquid
home-made soap

Food Control

Sometimes a sudden change in eating habits or a fixation on not eating, especially in young people, can be an indication of a lot of worries, fear or anger hidden below the surface. This gentle blend encourages breakthrough – so that troublesome emotions can surface. It also cools anger, so that these emotions can be looked at and dealt with calmly, and encourages the return of an appetite for life.

Benzoin 6 drops
Grapefruit 3 drops
Palmarosa 4 drops
30ml (1fl oz) of liquid
home-made soap

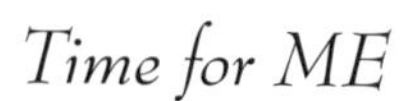

Time for ME

This blend is specially for those who have been knocked out for the count by viruses known or unknown and are taking a long time to recover. Don't give up! These beautiful ingredients will help to restore some of the energy you have lost, reduce anxiety and aches and pains, and leave you feeling, if not fully recovered, at least that the end of the tunnel is in sight.

Neroli 4 drops
Lemongrass 3 drops
Palmarosa 6 drops
30ml (1fl oz) of liquid
home-made soap

Stomach Soother

When you are regularly subjected to indigestion, constipation and/or diarrhoea, whether it be stress-related or as a result of something else, this blend will help soothe the spasms, reduce bloating and leave you feeling calm and worry-free.

Peppermint 6 drops
Neroli 3 drops
Roman Chamomile 4 drops
30ml (1fl oz) of liquid
home-made soap

Waterworks

Great for those who tend to get cystitis, this blend contains ingredients designed to reduce infection, swelling and pain, leaving you feeling a lot better.

Sandalwood 4 drops
Geranium 3 drops
Lavender 3 drops
Lemon 3 drops
30ml (1fl oz) of liquid
home-made soap

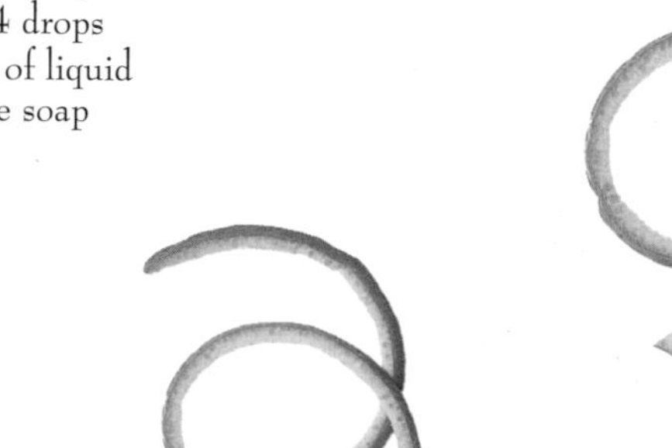

Glycerine soaps

The addition of glycerine to the basic white soap recipe results in a translucent effect to the end product. While the soap made in this way will never be completely clear, it does look wonderful, especially if you decide to colour it with plant products as suggested.

Glistening soaps are not the only benefits of using glycerine. Your skin will feel softer and younger, as glycerine reduces soap's tendency to dry out the skin.

One thing to note: you can expect the glycerine soaps to take fractionally longer to dry. As a result, I tend to make glycerine soaps in muffin tins or small moulds (just so I can enjoy them sooner).

Multiply the number of drops by 6 if you want to make one large batch, as on pages 50–51, instead of individual soaps in a muffin tin.

Zip

If you feel you lack get-up-and-go, you are feeling lethargic, have a few minor aches and pains and are generally unmotivated, try this blend. It will help to kickstart you into action, relieve those aches and pains, and leave you feeling fresh and clear-headed.

Ginger 3 drops
Vetiver 3 drops
Coriander 5 drops
Grapefruit 5 drops
30ml (1fl oz) of iquid
home-made soap

Ouch

This is great for those who are suffering after a hard workout – in the garden, the gym or the office. These oils are fantastic together as a blend for aching muscles and, since Rosemary isn't dominant in the blend, they will allow a restful night's sleep afterwards.

Marjoram 4 drops
Lavender 3 drops
Yarrow 5 drops
Rosemary 3 drops
30ml (1fl oz) of liquid
home-made soap

So Fresh

Invigorating, uplifting and excellent for the circulation, this blend will leave your skin tingling and your mind alert and ready for action. Definitely one to use in the mornings, it is also fantastic for relieving sinusitis, head colds and chest infections.

Rosemary 4 drops
Peppermint 3 drops
Marjoram 3 drops
Lemon 5 drops
30ml (1fl oz) of liquid
home-made soap

Gently Does It

Great for helping you recover from strained muscles or sprains, German Chamomile helps reduce swelling, Ginger helps heal bruises and Geranium is great for minor cuts and for clearing the skin.

Ginger 6 drops
German Chamomile 3 drops
Geranium 4 drops
30ml (1fl oz) of liquid
home-made soap

No More Tears

Something to dry the tears, calm you down and make you feel a bit more in control. This blend reduces anxiety, leaves you feeling more confident and is especially useful in relation to emotional or relationship issues. Neroli has the lovely effect of helping to restore your trust in the fact that things will work out for the best.

Neroli 4 drops
Sandalwood 4 drops
Patchouli 3 drops
Grapefruit 6 drops
30ml (1fl oz) of liquid
home-made soap

Addicted to Life

If you, or someone you love, is trying to recover from an addiction – whether it be coffee, food, alcohol, cigarettes or harder substances – this blend can help to relieve the cravings that are experienced during the recovery. They also help to encourage the liver to work more effectively to get rid of the toxins your body is trying to recover from.

Rose 6 drops
Vetiver 5 drops
Lemon 5 drops
30ml (1fl oz) of liquid
home-made soap

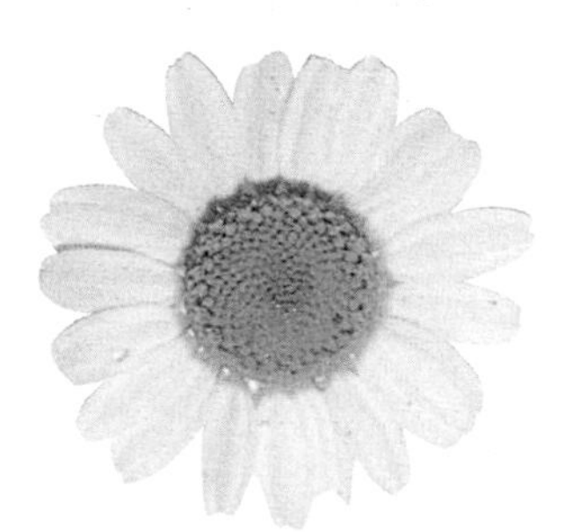

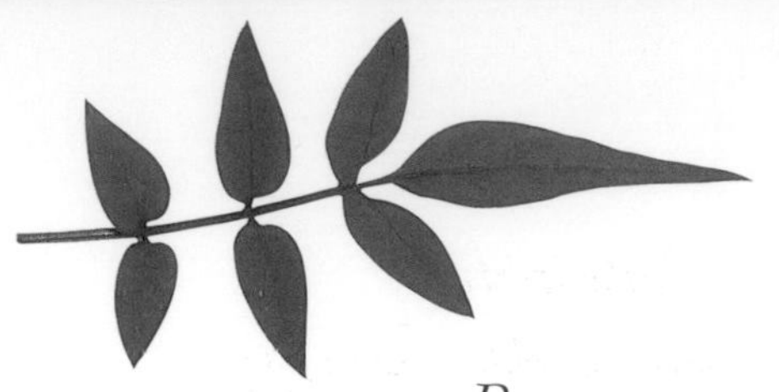

Fertility

If you are having difficulty conceiving, or want to encourage a menstrual cycle to regulate, this is an extremely successful blend. Try it in a massage oil as well for faster results. Some women using this blend have noticed an increased sensitivity to their bodies and have even felt ovulation occur – where they have been unaware of it previously.

Rose 3 drops
Vetiver 5 drops
Jasmine 3 drops
Grapefruit 3 drops
30ml (1fl oz) of liquid home-made soap

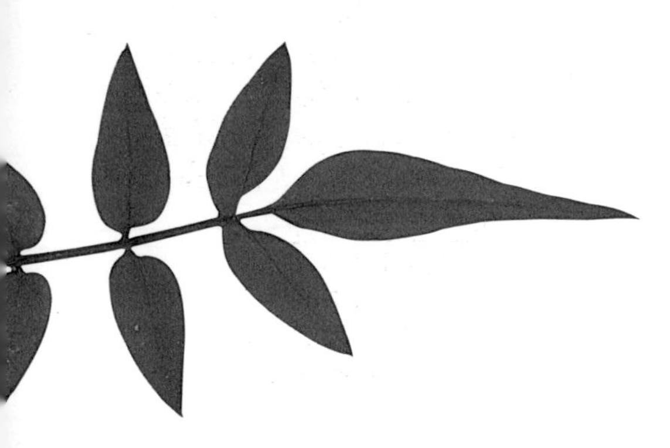

Moon Time

This is a luscious blend which helps to regulate menstrual cycles, leaves everyone feeling relaxed, aids insomnia and has a bit of an aphrodisiac effect.

Bergamot 5 drops
Jasmine 4 drops
Coriander 4 drops
30ml (1fl oz) of liquid home-made soap

Best for Breasts

This is wonderful for new mothers who are experiencing painful, swollen breasts and/or a lack of milk. Lemongrass encourages milk production, whilst the other ingredients help reduce pain and can ease the discomfort of cracked or sensitive nipples.

Roman Chamomile 4 drops
Lavender 3 drops
Grapefruit 3 drops
Lemongrass 4 drops
30ml (1fl oz) of liquid home-made soap

Back to Sleep

The ultimate cure for insomnia, especially in young children. This sweet blend reduces anxiety and encourages pleasant dreams.

Benzoin 4 drops
Neroli 4 drops
Roman Chamomile 3 drops
30ml (1fl oz) of liquid home-made soap

Dry Bedclothes

Anxious young children who are learning bladder control may benefit from this blend. Benzoin and Neroli take the stress out of the situation, whilst the astringent and toning effects of Grapefruit help in a mild way to strengthen the sphincter muscles in question.

Grapefruit 3 drops
Benzoin 5 drops
Neroli 3 drops
30ml (1fl oz) of liquid home-made soap

Romeo

Some young men go through a stage of applying so much cologne that the object of their affections runs the risk of being asphyxiated at 50 paces. This blend is designed to inspire confidence in the wearer, to clear his skin, boost his immune system and relieve muscle tension. It is also very subtle and fresh and contains key ingredients found in some of the commercial products that Romeo would like.

Vetiver 5 drops
Sandalwood 4 drops
Rosewood 4 drops
Orange 3 drops
30ml (1fl oz) of liquid home-made soap

Teenage Traumas

This blend is fantastic to have around the house when you are faced with young people brimming with hormones, bristling with aggression and trying hard to work out who they are. The blend helps clear the air, calms all household members and allows clear communication lines to be re-established. It's also good for nightmares and insomnia, especially in small children.

Benzoin 4 drops
Grapefruit 3 drops
Coriander 3 drops
Palmarosa 4 drops
30ml (1fl oz) of liquid home-made soap

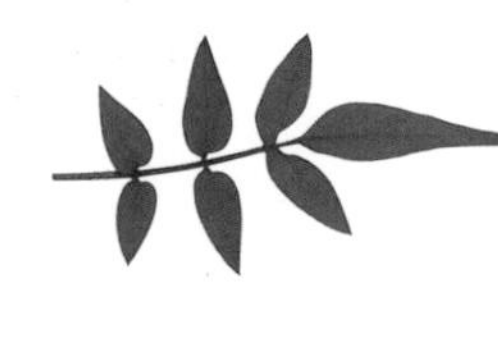

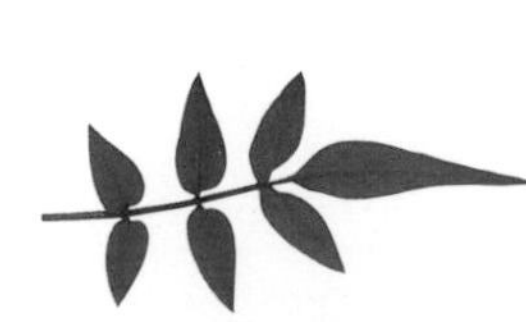

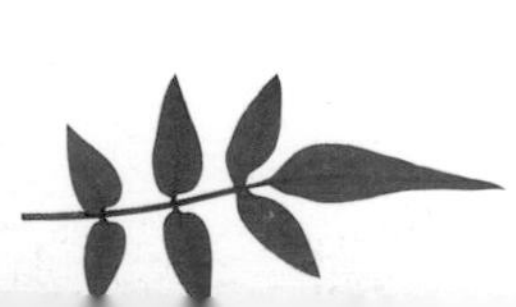

Anticipation

If you have something exciting to look forward to, this blend will help you to prepare for it. Roman Chamomile will keep you relaxed and calm the butterflies. Rosewood and Petitgrain will keep your skin rosy and clear, and Grapefruit will give your immune system a boost, so you don't have any last minute ailments to keep you from the ball.

Rosewood 4 drops
Petitgrain 4 drops
Roman Chamomile 3 drops
Grapefruit 5 drops
30ml (1fl oz) of liquid home-made soap

Readiness

This blend is very useful if you are experiencing a sense of foreboding, or feeling fearful, but are determined to be ready for whatever it is that life is going to throw at you. It leaves your mind clear, you'll feel very grounded and will be able to face the problem with strength and serenity.

Patchouli 4 drops
Frankincense 5 drops
Bergamot 3 drops
Neroli 3 drops
30ml (1fl oz) of liquid home-made soap

Moving On

It's time to say goodbye to a place, time, habit or person. Moving On helps to ease the pain involved in changing your life, giving you a bit of reassurance and the strength to pick yourself up and step into the future.

Rose 3 drops
Neroli 3 drops
Ginger 2 drops
Frankincense 5 drops
30ml (1fl oz) of liquid home-made soap

Pendulum

If you experience sudden mood swings and would like to feel calmer, more balanced and generally uplifted, try this blend. It's also absolutely lovely for mild skin conditions or if you would like to reduce fine lines and wrinkles.

Frankincense 5 drops
Neroli 4 drops
Rosewood 4 drops
30ml (1fl oz) of liquid home-made soap

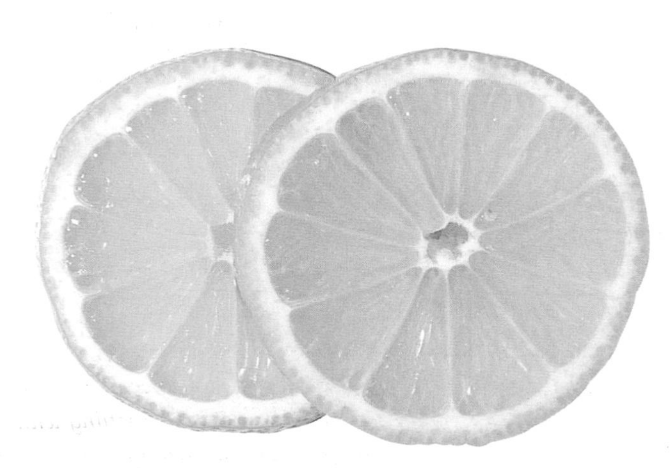

Hot Stuff

Hot flushes are no fun – even if you were hot stuff to begin with, the sudden temperature swings leave a lot to be desired. Try this blend to help cool you down and rebalance the hormones that are causing the swings.

Peppermint 3 drops
Palmarosa 3 drops
Rose 3 drops
Roman Chamomile 4 drops
30ml (1fl oz) of liquid home-made soap

The Fan Fights Back

When things are hitting you from all directions, this blend will help you to stand tall and firm and not make a drama out of a crisis. It also relieves muscular aches and pains, indigestion, nervous diarrhoea and tight-chestedness.

Neroli 3 drops
Vetiver 4 drops
Ginger 3 drops
Benzoin 5 drops
30ml (1fl oz) of liquid home-made soap

Dry Nights

This is wonderful for cooling the skin and reducing night sweats that result from hormone fluctuations. They are also gentle sedatives to help you to recover some of your sleep.

Lemon 4 drops
Palmarosa 3 drops
Rosewood 3 drops
Sandalwood 3 drops
30ml (1fl oz) of liquid home-made soap

Index by Symptom

Aromatherapy is a holistic therapy: rather than 'curing' specific medical conditions, it helps the body to regain its natural balance. In this way it improves general health, and can help to ease many minor conditions affecting the mind, body and spirit. The oils used in the recipes in this book have been specially chosen for their versatility and effectiveness. You may like to use the following guide when deciding which recipes to choose. As long as you follow the health and safety advice and stick to the recommended doses, making your own Aromatherapy products can be a delicious and satisfying way to improve your mental, physical and spiritual well-being.

	R Chamomile	G Chamomile	Geranium	Jasmine	Lavender	Neroli	Rose	Benzoin	Frankincense	Cedarwood	Sandalwood	Rosewood	Lemongrass	Patchouli	Palmarosa	Ginger	Vetiver	Grapefruit	Bergamot	Orange	Lemon	Peppermint	Rosemary	Yarrow	Marjoram	Coriander
acne		●	●		●	●	●			●	●	●					●	●	●		●		●	●		
anxiety	●		●	●	●	●	●		●		●	●		●	●	●	●	●	●	●	●			●	●	●
asthma					●			●	●	●	●										●			●	●	
athlete's foot			●		●							●		●			●				●					
bloating	●	●	●		●	●		●	●					●		●		●	●	●	●	●	●	●	●	●
bronchitis		●	●		●			●	●	●	●	●							●		●		●	●	●	
bruises		●			●											●								●		
catarrh				●	●			●	●	●	●							●			●	●	●		●	
cellulite			●		●								●					●			●		●			●
chapped skin		●	●		●	●	●	●	●		●	●		●			●	●	●					●		
constipation		●			●			●	●	●	●	●							●		●		●	●	●	
coughs				●	●			●	●	●	●	●									●	●	●	●	●	
cracked skin		●	●		●		●	●	●		●	●		●			●	●	●					●		
cystitis		●		●	●			●		●	●				●				●					●		
dandruff					●					●	●	●											●			
depression	●		●	●	●	●	●				●	●	●	●	●	●	●	●	●	●	●	●		●	●	●
dermatitis		●	●		●		●			●	●	●		●			●		●		●			●		
diarrhoea			●	●	●									●				●			●	●		●	●	

	R Chamomile	G Chamomile	Geranium	Jasmine	Lavender	Neroli	Rose	Benzoin	Frankincense	Cedarwood	Sandalwood	Rosewood	Lemongrass	Patchouli	Palmarosa	Ginger	Vetiver	Grapefruit	Bergamot	Orange	Lemon	Peppermint	Rosemary	Yarrow	Marjoram	Coriander
eczema	●	●			●			●		●	●	●		●					●					●		
excessive sweating			●										●		●						●					
gout	●																							●		
headaches	●	●	●		●									●							●			●	●	
healing wounds					●		●	●	●	●				●					●							
infections					●			●	●		●		●		●			●	●		●		●	●	●	
inflammation		●			●																			●	●	
insomnia	●	●		●	●	●	●	●			●	●		●			●	●	●	●				●	●	●
irregular periods		●	●	●	●	●	●										●	●	●					●		●
laryngitis		●		●	●			●	●		●	●										●	●	●		
lethargy				●		●		●		●			●	●		●	●				●	●	●		●	
menopausal symptoms		●	●			●											●									
migraine	●	●			●									●							●			●	●	●
mosquitoes					●					●			●	●	●		●									
muscular aches													●				●						●	●	●	
nausea		●	●		●	●								●	●	●		●	●	●	●	●		●		●
nervous tension	●	●	●	●	●	●	●		●	●	●	●	●	●	●	●	●	●	●	●	●			●	●	●
neuralgia	●				●				●				●											●	●	●
oedema			●		●								●					●			●	●	●			●
pain relief	●	●			●				●				●			●	●					●	●	●	●	●
painful periods		●	●	●	●	●	●		●								●		●		●			●	●	●
poor appetite			●			●		●					●	●	●	●	●	●	●	●	●	●	●	●	●	
poor concentration										●			●								●	●	●			●
pre-menstrual tension		●	●	●	●	●	●		●								●		●					●	●	●
psoriasis		●	●		●		●			●	●	●		●			●		●		●			●		
restlessness	●	●	●	●	●	●	●		●		●	●		●	●	●	●	●	●	●		●		●	●	●
rheumatic pain	●	●			●			●	●				●			●	●					●	●	●	●	●
sinusitis					●				●												●	●				
sprains					●											●	●						●	●		
strains					●											●	●						●	●	●	
stretch marks					●		●					●		●			●	●								
tight chest					●		●	●	●	●	●												●		●	
traumatic hair loss					●		●			●	●	●											●			
vomiting	●	●	●		●									●		●					●					
wheezing					●			●	●	●	●	●									●	●	●	●	●	

Index